THE GRAYWOLF MEMOIR SERIES

1991

DADDYBOY

A Memoir

Carol Wolfe Konek

To Thilla —
Thank you for keeping
the family history alive
and for keeping the family
members connected by love.
Also, for always showing
me the way.

GRAYWOLF PRESS

Carol Wolfe Konek

Publication of this volume is made possible in part by a grant provided by the
Minnesota State Arts Board, through an appropriation by the Minnesota State
Legislature, and by a grant from the National Endowment for the Arts. Additional
support has been provided by the Jerome Foundation, the Northwest Area Foundation,
and other generous contributions from foundations, corporations, and individuals.
Graywolf Press is a member agency of United Arts, Saint Paul.

Published by
GRAYWOLF PRESS
2402 University Avenue, Suite 203
Saint Paul, Minnesota 55114
All rights reserved.

9 8 7 6 5 4 3 2

First Printing, 1991

Library of Congress Cataloging-in-Publication Data
Konek, Carol Wolfe.
Daddyboy : a memoir / by Carol Wolfe Konek.
p.   cm.
ISBN 1-55597-153-9
1. Wolfe, Leonard (Leonard Merwin)—Mental health.   2. Alzheimer's
disease—Patients—Kansas—Biography.   3. Alzheimer's disease—
—Patients—Family relationships.   I. Title.
RC523.K66   1991
362.1'96831—dc20   91-16252

FOR MOTHER, TOMMY, AND LINDA

WITH LOVE AND GRATITUDE

WHERE'S CAROL? Where can she have gone? I can't find my sugarplum, Carol. I've looked everywhere and I can't find Carol.

Why, here's a little girl under the table. What a pretty little girl. Whose little girl are you?

Daddy's girl.

Yes, Daddy's girl. You're Daddy's sugarplum. Who am I?

Daddyboy. My Daddyboy.

He asks Mother, "How will we go home?" She replies, "We are home. This is where we live."

He turns away in disgust. Later, as though he has not been rebuked, he asks, "Will we take the train?"

She can't lie, won't play. "We're having a salmon and cheese casserole for dinner."

"Oh, goody."

She turns from her husband, weeping.

IT IS 1965 when Daddy's bike skids on gravel as he goes down a steep hill. He catapults over the handle bars, striking the curb with enough force to dent his helmet. He is treated for a broken collarbone and for deep lacerations on his legs, and sent home with the assurance that the helmet saved him from severe, possibly fatal head injury. Six months later, he complains to Mother that he has trouble recalling the names of his students, that he becomes confused in the middle of working out problems on the blackboard, and that he has run into the curb more than once while driving. Despite his awareness of his symptoms, he has refused to see a doctor, and has insisted on climbing up on the roof to repair rain-damaged shingles.

I receive several phone calls from Mother during which she whispers her concern while he is in the next room. "He's not himself. There's something odd about him. He forgets. He's silent. He stumbles. You know his memory. His coordination. It's not right. I tell him it might be a complication from the bicycle accident. He says nothing can be done for most brain injuries. Once, when I got cross, he said he thought he had suffered a stroke. That a doctor would not be able to do a thing... "

I respond, as I have a habit of doing, with advice. "You must take him to the doctor. If he absolutely refuses to go, call the doctor and tell him what you told me. Then tell Daddy the doctor called for him to come in for his post-accident checkup."

When I call the next weekend, her voice is hollow. "He's had tests. There will be more. It doesn't look good."

"I'll be right there." And I find myself waiting for her to dismiss my sense of urgency.

"Call me when you know your flight time."

The flight to California seems endless. I quell my sense of urgency by reciting "do not go gentle into that good night" to the rolling thunderheads beneath me, while resisting unwelcome memories of old hurts and unresolved conflicts.

I have hardened my heart against him. I have fought him, despised him, rejected him, and rebelled against everything he stood for. His peril forces me to complete the circle, to remember the adoration beneath the adolescent conflict which I recall.

I ENTER the hospital room through a sliding glass door from the sun-flooded patio, seeking him out in the shadows.

"Hi, Sugarplum."

The circle closes itself. Inside, there is only what is primary and essential and true. He is small. He is as fragile as... a man. All along, the tyrant, the giant, the judge was only Daddy.

I'LL HAVE TO perform more tests to confirm this diagnosis, but we are all but absolutely certain that we are dealing with a large, fast-growing tumor too close to the speech center and to other vital areas to be operable. What we are looking at is almost certainly a large, inoperable, malignant tumor of the brain." His eyes dart, momentarily, from the spot on the wall above our heads, to our faces—Tommy's, Linda's, Mother's, then mine.

"We'll be able to tell you more tomorrow. If I were you, I would prepare for the worst." He turns to leave the room, and then, over his shoulder, quietly says, "I'm sorry."

Linda and Mother lean into each other as though they can protect each other from the words of the doctor. Tom, true to his father's example and to his professional background, begins to reevaluate symptoms, dismissing the doctor's grim prognosis.

Tom spends the night reviewing the literature in the medical library. The next day, he tells us Daddy's symptoms are those of a subdural hematoma. When the doctor calls us together, proud of the reprieve his x-rays have provided, he announces with relief, "Your father has a subdural hematoma."

Daddy is prepared for surgery after being told the wonderful news. He beams at the story of Tom, the dentist, outdiagnosing the neurosurgeon. It is a family tradition that we can solve any problem given enough library time. We have been told all our lives that "few doctors are trained in science. Most medical training is the worst assortment of folk tales and superstition." Daddy believed that anyone who could read an instruction manual could learn to play the accordion or to diagnose brain ailments.

Still, we are grateful when the surgeon emerges from the operating room and tells us, "It was large, causing a great deal of pressure on the brain." He holds the palms of his hands together to illustrate. "When we drilled the hole in the skull, that old blood, about the consistency of crankcase oil, shot out with such force, it splattered the ceiling. You almost never see anyone go six months after an accident without exhibiting more pronounced symptoms than he had. Now we have to wait to see how the brain heals itself. It has to move back into the space the hematoma occupied. We have to see how many of the symptoms disappear, and how much permanent damage there is. Sometimes we get quite a bit of recovery, but, as I say, we're usually doing this kind of surgery six weeks rather than six months after the injury. This is most unusual."

Tom is ready to press his advantage with a doctor who was, after all, wrong. "Are you sure you're not being unduly pessimistic? Couldn't he be as good as new?"

The neurologist, always conservative, hedges. "I would be surprised to see him free of residual damage."

And, characteristically, over his shoulder, his parting words instruct us, "Let's count our blessings. He's going to live."

DADDY IS A MAN who distances himself from the moment with a camera. His part in a gathering is to record it in photographs which he develops in his darkroom, and hangs on hangers in the bathroom. He surrounds himself with light meters, tripods, still cameras, movie cameras, reflecting lights, musty leather camera cases, projectors, and viewing screens.

He captures my first bath after my home birth on an eight-millimeter movie. This documentary becomes a part of family reunion ritual until the younger, hospital-delivered cousins protest out of boredom and jealousy.

He creates reality as he directs and photographs us. I learn to pose. I learn that my every act is fascinating. I anticipate the vision of myself on the screen, even as I fall off my trike, twirl in my new dress, drink from the garden hose, or clutch Tommy's hand while squinting into the sunshine.

I develop a sense of audience before I develop a sense of self. And the audience is Daddy. I will never know if I would have been less conscious of his perception of me had he not shown me reels and reels of myself. As it was, I learned to see myself through his eyes, and to think of my life in photographic frames.

I THINK YOU KNOW how concerned I am about your father. Have I told you about how often he has nightmares? How he wakes me up, screaming at the top of his lungs, and how he leaps out of bed, frightened, unable to awaken?"

I wake with my heart pounding. Waiting for the night-shattering shout to repeat itself, and knowing as soon as it has, that it is Daddy's voice, shouting, "Help, help!" Running to their room, I find Mama holding Daddy in her arms. She is saying, "There, there," and he is crying, crying. Then he is saying, "Honey, don't be afraid. Daddy had a scary dream. A nightmare. I thought a bear was chasing me, but I was only dreaming. It was only make-believe. You mustn't be afraid."

Mother continues, "He frightened me last night as he has never frightened me before. He let out a scream, stood up and charged across the bed, and went to the corner where he was kicking the sliding glass door. He was hallucinating. He told me later he was protecting me from a tiger. But even when he kicked the glass door, and you know how much that must have hurt, he didn't stop. He didn't wake up. He was a wild man. His eyes were open. He kept shouting. It was horrible. I kept shouting, 'Leonard, wake up! You're dreaming.' And he wouldn't wake up."

"Oh, no." I begin to comprehend.

"Then he stopped in his tracks. He looked at me as though he were himself again. He said, 'I was dreaming that a tiger was attacking you.' Then he looked down, and we both saw that his foot was bleeding. He had broken the glass and cut his foot. We wrapped it in a towel and I took him to the emergency room. I think he's really worried about himself. He has been silent and distracted all day. I can't get him to discuss it."

"Do you think the nightmares are a result of his surgery? I know it has been years since the subdural hematoma, but what does the doctor say?"

"The doctor suggested that he take sleeping pills, but you know how Leonard is about medicine. He said they only made him groggy, and he didn't think they reduced the frequency of the nightmares."

"He has always been an active dreamer."

"But it was more than a dream. He didn't wake up as one does from a dream. It was as though he was possessed. He had become someone else. He was in a different world."

"Please, please, call the doctor."

"But what if there's nothing anyone can do? What if this is going to get worse and worse? I'm afraid to sleep with him. Ever since he kicked me in his sleep a few months ago, I've been afraid. I can't sleep soundly."

"Perhaps you should sleep in separate rooms," I venture, knowing full well that she won't accept my suggestion.

"Yes, I think you're right." Only now do I know that something is radically wrong. Only now do I begin to understand the depth of Mother's concern. She is a woman who underestimates the potential for conflict; she procrastinates, trivializes, ignores. She is a farmer at heart, a person who waits for the weather to change, for the crop to yield, for something outside herself to happen.

*A*ND THE SAND PILE *is my little town. Each ant has its own room, and its speck to carry. There, you carry your speck. Follow your brother. Like so. Follow the leader. Carry your specks to make a house. Just so. If I am an ant, there is a big person watching me thinking,* *why, she is only an ant. She thinks she is a girl, but she's an ant. She can follow the leader.*

"Ah. Ouch. Oh, no. Daddy. Daaaddy. Daaaddy."

His hands are swarming me, stinging me with sparks. I am a sparkler making sparks. Sparks go under my skin. He rips the straps of my sunsuit. Buttons fly like sparks. I burn bare in noon sun. Sweat mingles with tears. Mud rivers run down my tummy. He tears off his shirt and wraps it around me. He carries me like a baby. Crybaby. I am polka-dotted with welts. His tears sting my raw skin.

H ELLO. HELLO? HELLO." The silence on the other end of the line is compelling. It is morning on New Year's Day. An odd time for a prank call. I delay hanging up. "Hello. Who is calling, please?" I demand.

I strain to hear words wrapped in a hesitant whisper. "Leonard Wolfe. This is your father, Leonard Wolfe."

"Daddy. Daddy." I am confused. "Where are you, Daddy? What's wrong?"

"I'm here. At the airport."

"Here? At the airport? When did you arrive?" Even to me, my voice sounds too harsh.

After a long pause, he whispers in a faltering voice, "I don't know. Yesterday, I think."

"You came yesterday? Where is Mother? You came alone?"

"Yes. Alone. To take care of Dad's business. To help settle the business."

The family has been involved in negotiations to sell the family car dealership. My Uncle Benny has been making frequent calls to discuss the terms with my parents. Now I grasp the implications of Daddy's having flown to Kansas alone to work on the sale. He sat in the airport all night, unable to reach me, and unable to figure out how to find a cab.

"Daddy. I'll be right there. Promise me you'll just wait. Don't go outside. Wait right where you are. I'm coming."

When I reach the airport, I double-park in a loading zone, leave the car with the motor running, and race to find him, fearing that he may not be where I told him to wait. I search the faces of the travelers in the luggage area, but he is nowhere to be found. Gradually, he materializes in the person of a stranger.

He is small, diminished by the blue down jacket and black knit cap, and by the backpack he carries. His face is empty of fear. He waits patiently, the specter of a childhood self. A boy dressed for an outing, waiting for the scoutmaster and the other boys, lost in reverie, rehearsing the hike, dreaming the climb. For a moment, he becomes to me a grotesque lost child, somehow existing beyond me in time. Not my father.

"Daddy. Here I am. It's me. Oh, Daddy." He resists my embrace.

"Why didn't you let me know you were coming?"

"We didn't think it would be necessary."

"When I didn't answer the phone, did you think to get a cab?"

"I didn't know . . . I forgot your address." He falters, then regains his assured persona. "I was fine. I knew you would answer sometime."

I wonder how long he waited in the terminal, unable to call, unable to remember, unable to ask for help. I think of my New Year's Eve celebration and of his waiting, bundled up in his adventurer's gear, lost and too frightened to call out to another traveler.

I drive him home, plotting how I can keep the rest of the family from seeing what I have seen.

"I can drive you to Meade, Dad. I can take you to the family business meeting."

"I would appreciate that, Carol," he responds with a formality which allows me welcome distance. "You need to understand these business transactions." And, then, the telling concession – "And I need your advice. I need your help in making this deal."

During the week of negotiations, we are a team. I convey my interpretation of Daddy's ideas to Grandad, his brother Benny, and his sister Willa. He has held intellectual and economic dominance in this family alliance all of his adult life by confronting the sometimes tyrannical behavior of his father, bridging the distance between his father and his younger siblings, using his extensive knowledge of tax laws, economic principles, and profit-and-loss statements to ensure the survival of the business.

Now it is time to sell. Grandad is furious. He accuses Nana of plotting with the children to steal the business, to rob him of his livelihood. We are all in this together. If we sell the business, we might as well kill him. I find myself moving into my father's role in surprising and subtle ways. I ask him questions intended to reassure Grandad. Sometimes he answers. When he doesn't answer, or when he loses his train of thought, I answer for him, or pick up the dropped stitch of his thought. The others are compliant, recognizing that my intrusions protect them from a truth they don't want to face.

We confront and comfort Grandad. 'We appeal to his business sense, to reason, to greed. We want him out of the business. We want out. He wants to pass it down to the children. He bargains to "step aside," to "turn it over to anyone in the family who will run it." His children are firm. He must permit them to sell it for him. As I play the shadow role of my father's persona, defying Grandad, that regal old tyrant, I see the parallel between my father's and grandfather's conflict with each other and my lifelong struggle with Daddy. And how bitter I am to know that he is now too weak to stand firm against my will.

I T IS 1980, and after many telephone conversations with my mother in California, I have persuaded her to come to Kansas to check Daddy into a hospital for neurological tests.

Mother asks Daddy, "What kind of tests did the doctors do today?"

He studies the wall for an answer. We wait. "An EEG, I think...
Yes, an electroencephalogram."

"And what did the neurologist say when he examined your
eyes?"

He hesitates again, but remembers more quickly. He is on
track, his voice authoritative in the tone he uses for scientific dis-
course. "There's deterioration in the nerves. The kind they see in
Parkinson's disease."

If we name it, we can cope with it, master it, confront it. We can
choose our responses. We can seek a cure, or lapse into denial.

I avoid thinking of the distant future. "There is a treatment for
Parkinson's disease. L-dopa." Ugly name, L-dopa. The dope. An
idiot. Cruel joke. Impotence is a side effect. He has smuggled cop-
ies of *Playboy* into his hospital bag. On the nightstand is a copy
open to the centerfold.

He shifts attention from the diagnosis to his recent gift to me.
"What do you think of Santa Claus?" He speaks with a gentle, I-
am-as-before inflection, his face soft, seeking.

"I don't know what to say. You've given me so much. I'm not
sure I should let you buy me a car." My voice catches. Now is the
time to accept what he gives me, to let him give me a gift that is tangible and essential. Still, I need to deny my dependency.

Mother watches the television above our heads, silent tears rolling down her cheeks. Daddy and I carry on a conversation, our
topics and voices controlled, honoring the family code. Be strong
for the others. We discuss the food, the nurses' idiosyncrasies. I
talk. He agrees.

We stall in the moment. He will not be himself anymore. Every
day he will be less himself. Every day he will become less intentional. What has been voluntary will be replaced with what is
involuntary. Dis-ease of the central nervous system. Unease.
Anti-ease.

He always controlled every aspect of his being and of ours. He

learned how everything worked. He memorized formulas, quanti-
fied nature's laws, analyzed force, measured light, counted time
and motion, harnessed all the forces. He was a scientist whose in-
tolerance for magic obliterated mystery. The limits of knowing
were merely attributable to the limits of systems, of language, of
the evolution of understanding. We could discipline ourselves to
conquer the unknown. He would lead the way, a model of dedica-
tion to the life of the mind, to the rational life lived responsibly.

But he was not always with us. He studied mathematical puz-
zles written on scraps of paper, diverting his attention from the
gathered clan, sneaking furtive glances at problems while the rest
of us talked and laughed in the moment. Everything abstract or
philosophical was assigned to Leonard.

*M*AMA HAS A SURPRISE *for Carol. Come see your very
own baby brother. Now you are our big girl. You can help Mama
take care of baby Tommy. Mama has a baby boy. Daddy has a big girl.*
   Who are you?
   I am your Daddy.
   Who am I?
   You are my sugarplum. You are my big girl.
   Who are you?
   I am your Daddy.
   My Daddyboy?
   Your Daddyboy.

*W*E MEET FOR A CONFERENCE with the neurolo-
gist. He is austere, possibly disconcerted by the inclusion
of the patient in our conference. Daddy has reviewed his symptoms and made notes on his intellectual and physical deterioration
since the bicycle accident fifteen years ago. The neurologist may

not appreciate our deference to Daddy's interest in and knowledge of his medical status, but Mother and his brother Benny and I have nevertheless elected to include him in our discussion. He is, after all, the same person who discussed the disposition of his own remains when he was given a mistakenly bleak prognosis after the bicycle accident fifteen years ago. "You must not have a funeral. If people want to contribute to a memorial, ask them to send their money to the Vietcong." I recall the surge of pleasure it gave me to see that he could face his mortality, that his radical politics held firm when he was told he probably had an inoperable malignant brain tumor.

The neurologist reports the results of the tests. "The EEG is diffusely abnormal, indicating a general neurological defect. The CAT scan indicates mild cortical atrophy. The psychological tests, selected because they are specific for organically disturbed functions, show a marked decrease in short-term memory and some decrease in general intellectual functioning."

I am angry. I know he has discounted our assessment of Daddy's extraordinary intellectual abilities, and that what he calls "some decrease in intellectual functioning" is in reality a radical loss. I concentrate on my note-taking assignment as my uncle and mother cross-examine the doctor and Daddy stares into space, no longer attentive.

THE PHOTO ALBUMS are worn from children looking for answers to formal questions such as, "Who were you when you were a boy?," and, "Where was I born?", and "Remember when I was a baby?"

He has camera cases and light meters hanging on his shoulders. He sets up lights with moon-shaped reflectors whenever an occasion is significant. He lets his food grow cold on his plate as he focuses his movie camera on each person at the long, feast-laden table. His gifts remain un-

opened as he captures each child's look of delight with every gift. Nana
smiles in spite of herself, then covers her mouth with her hand, and turns
away while Grandad, encircling her waist with his arm, flirts with the
camera. Norman sweeps Hazel back into a Valentino embrace. Benny
tap-dances in the hall. Willa twirls with the awkwardness of a girl whose
baton is brand-new. The black-and-white movies evoke the glow of the
firelight, the fragrance of the pine on the mantle, the reflection of snow
falling in the yard beyond the windows where candles burn.

It is as though he coaxes the growth of the children and the changing of
the seasons with his camera. He is a man given to silence and understate-
ment, a man reluctant to praise or to demonstrate feeling. Yet he is a man
who records a loving vision of a family making rituals over time. He is a
man whose gift to his family is history.

M Y H U S B A N D J O H N mixes the salad. Mother boils potatoes for "real mashed potatoes." My daughter Jana sets the
table. Daddy hovers in our midst, wishing, I surmise, to be included, to be helpful.

"Daddy, why don't you go to the basement to get some chocolate ice cream from the freezer?"

My voice is too motherly as I offer him the double treat of helping and of being rewarded with ice cream for dessert. He beams,
shuffling toward the hall.

We are all seated before we miss him. I rush downstairs. He
stands in the middle of the laundry room, empty-handed. "I can't
find where the car is parked. How do you get out of this garage?" I
lead him upstairs, forgetting the ice cream.

We sit down at the table as the food is being passed. When the
salad is passed to him, he serves himself with the large salad serv-
ing fork. He keeps it and eats the remainder of his meal with the
large, unwieldy fork. No one points out his error. We chatter too
brightly, filling the empty space left by our mutual sense of loss.

I T IS 1980, prior to the acknowledgment in medical journals and the press of the epidemic of Alzheimer's disease. The neurologist notes the shortened gait, the hand tremors, and the occasional mask-like appearance of Daddy's face, and concludes that we are probably dealing with Parkinson's dementia syndrome – a progressive, degenerative brain disorder which will allow a life span of approximately ten years more. We should have met privately with the doctor. Daddy should not be hearing this. I should not have insisted on the examination by a specialist. Guilt protects me from sorrow.

This is the first of many discussions with neurologists. The family will always leave such consultations to mull over unanswered or unasked questions. We will, on each occasion, gain additional insights into the ways we shield ourselves with selective perception. Mother and Benny and I each heard the prognosis differently. We only speculate about what Daddy heard, or what he made of what he heard. Mother, who is plain-spoken to a fault, will continue to voice her questions and observations to the man who has made virtually every decision affecting her life since she was his twenty-year-old bride. She will, like many women of her generation, be liberated by abandonment and despair.

M OTHER, DADDY, AND I sit at my kitchen table after he has checked out of the hospital. Mother and I search for small-talk topics. He has never been one for small talk. "Get a sheet of paper, Carol. You must write down some financial information." He proceeds to list the details of his finances with clarity and precision, admonishing me that my mother is never to invest in real estate, a familiar cardinal rule.

I ask good questions, rising to the occasion of being taken into the male circle of financial discussion. My mother is outside the circle. I realize that I betray her in allowing her exclusion. Yet, there is something exhilarating about his soliciting my attention. How often I have thrilled to the shifting balance of power in this intimate triangle. How often we have excluded Mother from decisions.

WHY, CAROL, *what are you doing in that crib? Give me those scissors! What's come over you? Give them to me, young lady! You could hurt the baby! What do you have to say for yourself?"*

"I fix Tommy's hair. Tommy needs a haircut."

I am across Daddy's knees, his hand searing sharper than ant stings, hotter than boiling oatmeal spilling on my arm, sharper than skinning my knee on the pavement.

"You must never, never, never, never come near the baby with scissors!"

I'm a bad girl. I'm not Daddy's girl anymore.

DADDY REFUSES to take off his down jacket and his knit cap. He is a guest at my kitchen table, where he sits bundled up like a child waiting for his mother to put on his snow boots, hypnotized by the promise of snow filling the yard.

I introduce him to friends who stop by, wanting to know him while there is time. He is courteous, remembering etiquette learned by rote in a distant time. I sometimes think I become the mother of his memories, signaling with my tone of voice that he is to pay attention to his manners. His presence is required.

He is in command of himself for the moment. "I am pleased to meet you," he says to my friend Marni.

She is tactful enough to make statements, rather than to ask questions demanding answers that might fall through the synaptic net. "I understand you're enjoying the Kansas weather."

"Yes. I enjoy the Kansas weather," he picks up the cue, smiling.

"Carol tells me you plan to visit her for several weeks."

"Yes. I am enjoying my visit." He studies her face, as though he feels her sympathy.

Then, he offers her a surprising gift. He has gathered photocopies of all of his articles on Alzheimer's disease in a manila envelope. "Would you like to read about my disease?" he asks politely, extending the envelope to her. "It is very interesting."

"Why, yes. Thank you." She sorts through the articles, her head down and her voice matter-of-fact, showing respect for his scientific objectivity.

He points to photographs of atrophied brain cells. He is deserted by his scientific vocabulary. "You can see what happens," he says.

A LONE IN MY HOUSE, I read old letters, entertaining myself with domestic rites during the blizzard I have awaited all winter. Sudden treasure. Letters from Mother to Daddy, saved, no doubt, by Nana, for whom each letter was a bit of the sacred now. Among the faded letters, I find courtship letters, a wedding certificate, a budget for their honeymoon at the Lore Locke Hotel in Dodge City, and a half-completed honeymoon letter from Mother to her mother.

Her letters brim with eagerness and anticipation. She is taking a course at Emporia State Teachers College to prepare her to teach in a one-room schoolhouse. She misses her fiancé. She is restrained in her expression of affection, but the emotion of the somewhat formal prose is apparent. I am a voyeur, looking into a kaleidoscope of the past.

The snow falls slowly outside my window. The flakes are huge. The kitchen has the magic, bright glow of light filtered through a veil of snow.

I find a tiny diary amidst the letters. Most of the pages are blank.

The pages are ruled into five sections. In my father's almost un-readable script are precious, one-sentence entries dated 1922. The eleven-year-old sees himself as an adventurer. "We strike out for California." "We cross the desert." And after the family has arrived in California, he conquers the territory of the unfamiliar. "Today I buried treasure." "Today I joined a club." "Today I buried secrets." "Today I fought with Homer. Licked him."

The gaze of the child in the photograph is serious. Leonard stands beside his brother Norman, his hand on the shoulder of the seated look-alike. The photograph predates their differentiation. They are dressed like perfect imitations of Little Lord Fauntleroy, in velvet jumpers with white blouses, white hose, and buckled shoes. Norman has yet to become the clown who will grow into a rebel. His brow is smooth. His eyes are serene. Later photographs will record his departure from the solemn dignity he now learns from the older brother who knows how to pose for the photographer.

In even later photographs, Leonard's gaze will remain constant. He will retain this childhood solemnity. Norman will grow more frantic, playing practical jokes the instant before the click of the shutter. He will be captured making devil's horns behind the head of his unsuspecting brother, sweeping his future wife Hazel into a dramatic backbend for a lascivious kiss, or posing unexpectedly as mimed sophisticates, playboys, gangsters, idiots.

Their mother will continue to dress them alike. Their father will give them the same lessons in outdoor survival, salesmanship, and religious orthodoxy. Yet, they will go off in their own directions. Norman will be the life of the party, desperate for attention until the day he takes his last drink, the drink that ends his life. Leonard will seek perfection and understanding until he gradually, day by day, cell by cell, loses his mind.

Now, there is only this precious trash. These letters, these photographs, this diary. This forgotten tin box.

IT IS ICY COLD in the morning. We don't turn up the heat because we're not made of money. Mama makes toast in the oven under the flames, then leaves the oven door open and backs up to the stove, enjoying the warmth.

"The holes are getting bigger. I'll wear out my socks," I whine, hating my own baby voice.

"What about the cardboard from yesterday?" Daddy asks.

"I wore through the cardboard." I try to sound grown up.

"Well, let's see if we have another cereal box." He takes two shredded-wheat biscuits from the box and places them in a jar.

"But it falls apart before I even get to school," I complain.

"Today, I'll give you two layers," he says.

Mother clears the table as Daddy draws around my foot on the side of a shredded-wheat box, whistling under his breath.

"She'll be comin' 'round the mountain when she comes."

7

MOTHER REPORTS that Daddy was very excited yesterday when she told him she was taking him out for dinner. He went down to the office and sorted through many drawers, searching, it finally became apparent, for his keys. Then he shuffled up the stairs, hanging onto the railing as he took trembling toehold after trembling toehold on the very edge of each stair.

The impulses from his brain to his feet lag. His eyes reveal his excitement, while his once-nimble feet falter. He wears the tattered remnants of half-remembered roles, putting on a second wristwatch over the one which has inexplicably stopped telling time. His hands wander over his chest and then his hips, searching for his misplaced wallet.

When she leads him out the door, down the front steps, and to the van, he asks cheerfully, "Shall I drive?" I invent, then erase from my mind, her response. Male roles of responsibility are symbolized in the watch, the keys, the wallet. Does he mourn the loss of the man, the person he was? Or does he ride along like a passive but anticipating child? Does she bribe him with ice cream so that he will give up the responsibility of driving, of opening her door for her, of reading the menu and asking her for her order?

E ACH SATURDAY, Mother and I talk for an hour or more. I have long since rationalized that my phone bill for California calls does not exceed the gasoline bill I would gladly pay could I drive across town to visit and help with the housework on a weekly basis.

We begin with the weather, the season, the children, the yard, the week, and then the day. Her weather is windy. The storms will move eastward. We will have thunderstorms and tornado warnings by Tuesday unless the rain dissipates over the Rockies. It is an unseasonably cool and wet spring. In my yard, bright purple and scarlet anemones surpass the hyacinths which this week bow sadly toward the damp earth. The redbud tree by the porch now scatters blossoms on the porch, the first pink petal shower of spring. Last week I regretted the fading of daffodils, but only because I had forgotten the advent of anemones.

She never stops marveling at the year-round California growing season. She is making soup and baking bread. She recites the prices of abundant fresh vegetables which simmer in soup on her stove as we talk. I tell her the per-pound price of each ingredient in my soup. I am connected to her by rituals as delicate as the scent of her bread in my mind.

We move cautiously toward the inevitable subject of Daddy's suffering and her endurance. Last week she reported that he was unable to unclench his fist. She reminded me that the doctor had warned that he would one day be perfectly rigid, his whole body clenched into a fetal fist. This week she does not mention his rigidity. I do not ask. She reminds me of an earlier conversation by remarking that his hallucinations have been less frequent and less prolonged. While he often appears to be watching something Mother does not see, he does not warn her of the danger posed by his demons.

She adds, as an afterthought, "He did have an imaginary visit from Benny this week. He laughed and laughed. When I asked him what was funny, he responded, 'That Benny. That Benny.'" I imagine him laughing at a secret joke told him by his poltergeist, his little brother Benny.

I am happy long after hanging up. If only he could now move into a new phase. If he could have the gift of visits with childhood playmates. If all the friends and family who loved him when he was a child could gather around him now, telling him jokes and stories, bringing him gifts and memories. If he could resurrect the loving parents, the ornery brothers, he could then surely remember his hikes in the grove, the hiding places of his secret treasures, the slow summer afternoons and their promise of cicadas and fireflies by evening.

DADDY OWNS only one suit. It is a suit he inherited from Grandfather Norman. It is gray worsted wool, with cuffs and elbows gleaming with wear. It has a full back, gathered onto a half belt. Grandfather Norman was a man with a sense of style, so the suit must have been elegant in its time, but no one can recall the year. It becomes the symbol of Daddy's rebellion. He wears the suit to the few obligatory funerals he cannot avoid. Because he has the suit, Nana invites him again and again to attend church. She would shudder at the word "atheist" were he to use it in her presence.

I am dressed in a costume of pink and green curled crepe paper. I am moved by the music "Jesus wants me for a sunbeam, a sunbeam, a sunbeam" and find myself twirling against the background chorus of flowers. As I twirl, I catch glimpses of his rising image. He is laden with

camera cases and light meters. Beneath the whirring motion picture cam-
era, his smile is brilliant. I am the star of his show. I am my Daddy's sun-
beam, his sunbeam, his sunbeam.

I ATTEND A CONFERENCE sponsored by the College of
Health-Related Professions for helping professionals who have
Alzheimer's patients in their charge. The conference, designed for
fifty professional participants, draws more than four hundred,
some of whom are family members of Alzheimer's victims. It is, as
the program chair concedes, "a season of high consciousness."
We testify to the "graying of America." We testify to the frustration, the confusion, the searching for meaning by caregivers.

I am angry before the neurologist begins his keynote address.
The audience consists of more than ninety-five percent women. I
prejudge the speaker. We will undoubtedly listen to a man assure
us of the redeeming features of caregiving. He is clinically precise,
with a forthright manner I associate with neurologists who, perhaps more than any of their peers, learn to accept and acknowledge
their own limitations and the mysteries of medical science.

He admonishes us to consider that the way in which a society
deals with the aged challenges the way it views humanity. We
must, as a society, come to terms with the fact that in the year 2020
there will be fifty-five million people over the age of sixty-five with
10 percent of the population over eighty and 5 percent over ninety-
five.

For a moment I experience a surge of hope. Perhaps he will address the political implications of the problem. Perhaps he will as-
sail national priorities.

The speaker moves on to the history of Alois Alzheimer's efforts
to distinguish dementing disease from previous psychological
definitions. Prior to Alzheimer's work in 1907, emotional and
physical diseases were not distinguished.

Using slides, the neurologist points out the physiological characteristics associated with the disease. He shows a normal brain in one frame, and an Alzheimer's victim's brain in another frame, pointing to the wider spaces between the convolutions in the diseased brain, then to the oddly clustered neurofibrillary tangles and irregularly deposited plaques which distinguish an Alzheimer's victim's brain. He describes slide after slide. Finally, he points to the degree of shrinkage which distinguishes the damaged from the normal brain. He acknowledges the difficulty in diagnosis, asserting that autopsy provides the only certain test. The CAT scan has its limitations, as does a test in which air is introduced into the spinal column. I take rapid notes, absorbed by the act of trying to include both sketches and text of the lecture.

The speaker outlines the progressive stages of the disease, categorizing them as the forgetful stage, the confusional stage, and the vegetative stage. The first stage is characterized by forgetfulness, verbal errors, and the blunting of conversational, perceptual, and cognitive abilities. During this stage, the victim will not always be himself, making errors of which he is aware. The victim is likely to be depressed and to exhibit denial. The second stage is marked by disorientation, wandering, rambling, and diminishment of social skills. The speaker explains that in this stage "the victim loses what makes him human," that qualities of mutuality, independence, interdependence, and responsiveness to others vanish. The speaker matter-of-factly assures us that in the vegetative stage the victim has no human capacity to interact, to reflect curiosity, to respond, or to feel.

The speaker sorts through the current theories on the cause of the disease, and then, painstakingly, discusses "cures" described in popular and yellow journals, and experiments reported in medical journals. He tells the audience that a cure, when it comes, will be widely publicized. He shatters our hope when he explains that none of us need worry that some doctor, somewhere, is curing Alzheimer's patients without our knowledge. We are not depriving those for whom we care the hope of a cure.

He counsels us to contemplate the theology of the dilemma in which we live. He commends us for investing in the care of another human being when there is so little response. He believes we exemplify the Easter season, and that "we are human when we give care when we cannot see any visible reward or response. We do it because it is our nature."

The neurologist is a religious man and a dedicated physician. He makes me furious. At the break, an acquaintance beams at me. "Isn't he wonderful? Don't you just love his way of looking at this?"

"Oh, do you have an Alzheimer's victim in your family?"

"Oh, no. I just came to learn more about the disease."

"I thought he gave a very good speech. He is very knowledgeable on the subject."

"But didn't you think it was inspiring?"

"No, I didn't. I don't appreciate a man who has never bathed or changed the diapers of another human being telling me about the redemption of caregiving."

She is shocked. I am ashamed of my bad manners, but I can't stop. I am trembling with anger.

"Every week when I talk to my mother on the phone, I hear of the costs of her self-sacrifice. If she needs to learn what it means to be human by giving up her life for someone the speaker describes as 'no longer human,' the God he describes is worse than crazy."

"Oh, I'm sorry . . . "

I still can't stop. "Doctors should ask caregivers how they endure, not tell them what their sacrifice means. And we need some attention to the personal and social costs of that care. If it is so sacred, why aren't teams of people in line to assist the caregiver? Why doesn't the government fund research and family assistance? It is irresponsible for a doctor to discuss the physiology of the disorder and to be so blasé, so naive, on the meaning of the suffering."

"I can see that you have given this a lot of thought." She tries to cut me off, embarrassed by my diatribe.

"And I can see that he has given precious little thought to the lives of women like my mother. A decade out of her life can teach her what it means to be human? What if she knew before she started? She is like a woman in an ancient culture, obediently leaping into the open grave of her husband. And her suicide is socially sanctioned. No one will lift a hand to stop her."

She seeks an escape. She assures me that "we must have lunch," that she is "eager to know more about the kind of support volunteers can give."

I wonder, as I return to my seat in the auditorium, if this rage will ever subside. I wonder if I will ever learn to smooth a surface of good manners over this surging pain.

Irene Bernside, a nurse who has written extensively on the subject of caring for demented patients, explains that the film, *Gramp,* will not be shown. The movie was made for the audience of caregivers. Its impact on victims of family members is potentially too devastating. While the conference was originally designed for caregivers, it has been expanded to meet the requests from family members. Alzheimer's disease must be confronted in stages. A person in the early phase of the disease would be plunged into depression if shown this movie, a portrayal of a victim in an advanced stage of the disease.

My point of view shifts to the victims in the audience. They have already heard too much. How horrible for them to view the slides documenting the shrinking of their brains, the widening valleys between the convolutions, the tangling of the nerves, the relentless formation of the plaques. I look around. If there are victims in the audience, their faces are masked with stoicism. They do not identify themselves with tears. No one in the audience betrays the inner devastation we all must feel.

Ms. Bernside has the subtle blend of toughness and gentleness characteristic of my favorite caregivers. She discusses four progressive stages of the disease, rather than three. She is more focused on the coping strategies of the caregivers than on the physiological, psychological, and social symptoms. She teaches the strategies of comfort and reassurance. She discusses the use of simple language, the use of visual and nonverbal reinforcement of meaning. She considers family members the experts on the manifestations of the disease in any given patient. While she has observed professionals who are threatened by the expertise of family members, she affirms the value of caregivers' understanding.

She pleads for a truce between family and professional caregivers who are often at odds over caregiving styles and strategies. It occurs to me that a spouse or child whose whole life has become centered on selfless caregiving must feel abandoned and superfluous when the victim is finally sent to a care home. The person who has sacrificed his or her life for the comfort and well-being of the victim gains no recognition from the victim, from society, or from the professional caregiver who takes over the responsibility with the calm assurance that the irrational behavior of the victim is within the realm of what is considered normal. The coolness of professionalism must strike the abandoned family caregiver as repudiation, as trivialization of the sacrifice around which one's whole world has evolved.

Ms. Bernside compares the clinical distinctions between depression and dementia. Dementia is characterized by impaired memory, diminished social skills, reduced self-awareness, and Sundowner's Syndrome (night wakefulness and daytime drowsiness), followed by delusions and then incontinence. Dementia reduces judgment, affect, memory, clarity, and orientation to place, time, and persons.

She intersperses this grim catalogue with anecdotes. She describes a patient who had been extremely agitated by the loss of his car prior to being placed in a care home. A nurse found him one night straddling the toilet, facing the wall, turning an invisible steering wheel and madly shifting gears by flushing the toilet over and over. She also tells of a patient, a military man with mechanical and technical as well as administrative abilities, who drove the entire staff of the care home mad with his ingenuity in hiding his feces. Finally, they discovered that he had disassembled the heating register to hide his cache.

Now there are tears on the faces of her listeners. She presses home her point. No caregivers, either family or professional, will survive without the ability to see the absurdity, the humor, the hilarity in the plight leading to madness and beyond. It is too grim a process to survive without the cultivation of a genuine sense of delight in the absurd.

Caregivers have the opportunity to understand the nature of human frailty as others may not. We can laugh or weep. We can laugh or perish.

For weeks, I laugh when I recall the image of the man driving his toilet. It is a redemptive laugh that I find much more comforting, much less infuriating, than the philosophical ruminations of the neurologist. It is an image worth the price of admission.

*W*E LIVE IN PLAINS, KANSAS, *where my daddy is boss at Grandad's car agency. We all must work together if we are to make it a success.*

Mother helps with the books. I sweep the floor after school. Some days I dust the oil cans and fan belts and windshield wipers and candy bars.

I never get to have candy or pop, because they will rot my teeth and provide no nutritional benefit, unlike peanuts which will keep me alive if I'm stranded on a mountain or in a blizzard on the highway. When I dust the candy shelves, I notice the candy bars aren't selling very well. We will probably have to throw them out.

I take a teeny-weeny bite from each corner of one candy bar each day after school, carefully spitting out the foil I get with each bit of delicious chocolate. I know it would be stealing to take one whole Hershey bar, even though Daddy probably wouldn't miss it.

He calls me into the back room, where Ned, the mechanic, can't hear. He is stern, with the muscle along his jaw quivering the way it does when he doesn't want to spank me. I have ruined more than half a box of Hershey bars. Whatever was I thinking of? Did I want our customers to buy germy candy? Did I want them to think we had mice? Did I want to ruin business? I am working at the Wolfe Motor Company as part of the family team. Our business is no better than our good name. We have to be honest, give good service, and sell good products so our customers can trust us. A ruined candy bar may seem like a small thing, but it is no different than selling a car with a cracked block or with an odometer that has been set back.

"You would deserve a spanking if this were not a business. I've talked to your mother, and we've decided to give you an opportunity to work off the company's loss. You will work every day after school for your usual five cents per hour until you have paid for one-half of a box of Hershey bars. That will be a total of sixty cents. You will come here directly after school until your debt is paid."

After this, everyone knows about me. Ned is sorry for me. The customers treat me like a baby. Daddy doesn't let me wait on customers while he is busy in the shop. I stop dusting the candy bars until a fine layer of dust tells customers business isn't so good.

E ACH DAY brings new confirmation of the bleak prognosis of Alzheimer's disease. We are a family accustomed to gathering to celebrate and separating to accept loss. We speak what we wish to acknowledge and deny what gives us pain. Like other families, our codes of behavior are well known but poorly articulated. Each of us pulls away from the others to mull over the memories we now know are only partly shared. Each of us blames the others when they voice private loss. We seek to tighten individual bonds before the final unraveling. We are angry at one another because we can't attack the disease. We are guilt-stricken. We are forgiving. Each of us seeks to be the most loved, the most essential part of a life being buried in shrinking and dying brain cells.

IT IS 1983 when I fly to California to help celebrate my parents' fiftieth wedding anniversary. Mother pulls up to the curb of the loading area. I toss my bags into the back of the van, and we enter the heavy stream of rush-hour traffic. She is at ease on the freeway, changing lanes abruptly and making colorful remarks aimed at the aggressive California drivers.

"He knows you're coming. He seemed excited. You know, I can tell when he is looking forward to something. I had quite a scare before I came to get you. I was cleaning the patio and picking up in the yard. He was trying to help. I thought he was behind me and turned around to speak to him, and he was gone. Well, he wasn't gone. I couldn't see him because he had fallen down, fallen over backward. He does that now, but he would do it anywhere. I have to let him walk around."

I agree, and she continues, "If he falls, I have to know he would fall even if he were in someone else's care, or if he were in a care home."

"What did you do?" I ask.

"I helped him get up. He took the longest time. I got a chair, helped him grasp it to use for leverage."

"But how did you pick him up?" I ask.

"I can't lift him. I told him, 'Now, you have to get up yourself. You know I can't lift you.'"

It is more than jet lag I feel when I come here. When last I saw him six months ago, he did not fall over backward. A fall would have been a crisis. Now I need to adjust to his falls as being normal incidents rather than crises.

The neighborhood contrasts darkly with the freeway we have

just left. I concentrate on street names and house numbers, trying not to picture his fallen, rigid body on the patio.

*G*RANDMA'S KITCHEN *is cool and bare. The forlorn lamb bleats in a wooden box by the black woodburning stove.*

Tommy and I take turns holding the baby bottle filled with cow's milk against the determined tug of the lamb's mouth. The lamb wobbles on fragile legs, pulling fiercely at the bottle.

I want the lamb for my very own. Please Daddy. Let us take him home.

No. Lambs need to live on the farm. They are not pets.

Oh, please, Daddy. We can keep it on the back porch.

No.

Then chickens. Baby chicks.

No.

Please, Daddy. Just two. One for Tommy. One for me.

Well. We'll see.

Oh, goody. Oh, Daddy. We'll take care of them. Won't we, Tommy?

You must take care of them. They are not playthings. They are living creatures.

We drive back to town with the chicks in a shoe box, scattered with chicken feed, and an extra sack for later.

Daddy connects a light bulb to an extension cord, and hangs the bulb through a hole cut out of a large cardboard box. We scatter grain around two jar lids of water. My chick is Cheep. Tommy's chick is Chirp. They are easy to tell apart. Cheep is brighter yellow than Chirp.

Tommy goes to sleep while I lie awake listening. His easy breathing assures me that I am the best mother to the chittering, skittering chicks.

I wake to silence. Then I am scared. I hurry to the porch where the light shines on two lifeless balls of yellow fluff.

Daddy is there in the middle of my scream. Naked. Furious.

I am twice shocked. The horror of the fragile, dead chicks. And his surprising, naked body, a secret revealed. Death and sex present themselves to me in the same instant.

M OTHER TAKES ME directly from the airport to the
meeting. The house and the hostess are California casual.
The people gathered for the Alzheimer's support-group meeting
chatter in groups of two and three, their faces lively, their voices
animated. The sense of dread I have locked in my chest since she
told me we would come to the meeting before going home dissolves as eager eyes seek me out and welcome me into the circle.

Rita, the hostess, is the tough, yet sensitive leader of the talk-
ative group. Everyone wants to talk at once. The women and
daughters and the sole man all came to talk. Rita tries to gauge the
needs of newcomers and regulars, to subtly instruct in the art of
balancing listening and talking. She is intense, her bright eyes
accustomed to probing beneath smooth surfaces. She calms the
aimless chatter and focuses the group's attention on a first-time
visitor, Anne, who has driven from another county to find this
meeting, after discovering that her neighborhood group had become inactive. She had attended only one of that group's meetings. She is sleek, tanned, elegantly dressed. Her eyes flash with
rage and humor.

"I felt like killing myself. I couldn't stay there. He wouldn't
wash his hair. Or bathe. My husband was a community leader. He
was involved in everything. The arts. Theater. All good causes. He
was a leader in the county's civil rights movement. He gave his
heart and soul to the community. Now he has. . . we have no one.
No one calls or comes around. We belong to a country club. Last
week one of those sanctimonious, curious women, a person I
hardly know, came up to me and said, 'Oh, Anne, what can I do?'
And I cried. I hated myself for crying in front of her. How can you
tell them what you want them to do? You want them to treat you as
though you are still alive. As though your life still matters. But
they can't. They don't call or come by or invite you out. I couldn't
ask her to have her husband call my husband.

"My husband won't admit there is anything wrong with him.
He's heard the diagnosis many times, yet he acts as though he is

still in charge. My son runs the business, but every day my husband goes to the office that they reserve for him. It's a shambles. No one could do anything in that office. But everyone he works with is courteous. They indulge him. They behave as though he still has a place, a role in the business.

"We've been through the turmoil of getting the car away from him. His license expired. He had to go for a test. He could answer only one question on the test. He failed it, naturally. Then he found a friend who took him to another town to take it. I found out the friend had taken the test for him. I called him and told him, 'If my husband has an accident, I will hold you responsible.' Now he stays away from my husband. I drove him off. I was furious, but now I wish I hadn't called. He was just helping my husband with his denial.

"We're isolated. I was no longer comfortable sharing a room with him. I got a condo with thirty-five hundred square feet, thinking we would have enough space; but that isn't enough space for someone like him. He tears everything apart. He denies his illness. He won't bathe. He has no judgment. We lived in a rental property for seven years while he told me prices would come down. When I bought this condominium, I hired a man to care for him, but nothing worked.

"I want to kill myself. I can't live in this tomb of his illness. I want my life. I have this life left to live." She pauses, and surveys the group for criticism. The women listen intently as she continues.

"I finally moved out. I took a one-room apartment, just took a few dishes with me, a few pans. But I can't be alone. I go home after work and look at the four walls. I'm married forty-two years. Nothing has prepared me to be alone. I don't know how to be alone or how to stop being alone. We're deserted by our couple friends. I can't go to bars. I want companionship, yet I don't know how to get it."

Anne stops suddenly, as though surprised by the force of her outpouring. Rita takes up the slack in the group tension. Her eyes pace from person to person. "What do you think about what you've heard? How can Anne find companionship? Why don't we tell her how we deal with the isolation of Alzheimer's disease?"

Sara glances at Anne, then studies the teapot on the table in front of her. "I'm totally alone. I've been totally alone for three years. He's there, and I take care of him, but he's not the person I knew. He's not responsive to me. He has no control over his functions. He messes everything. I shut the door to my room so that he won't ruin my carpet. He's ruined the rest of the house. His room has no carpet. I can just wipe up after him there."

Anne mentions an insurance policy that, for a premium of thirty dollars a month, pays twelve hundred dollars a month for care-home costs. Everyone scoffs. A serious white-haired woman says in a bureaucratic tone, "Medicare won't pay for custodial care designed to benefit the caregiver. Medicare does nothing to benefit or contribute to the convenience of the caregiver." Others nod.

The topic of companionship is abandoned. I wonder if Anne is being ignored because she's so obviously well-off. There are few other women in the room who could hire a man to drive and clean, enabling them to escape to a one-room apartment.

Sara continues, "It's really like caring for an animal. All you finally think about is the stench of excrement and urine. You think only of how to remove spots, how to outwit the pisser who pisses in every corner."

Ruby, who has been remote until this point, adds, "You stand there and plead with him to go. And he won't. You give up pleading and then he does. But not in the toilet or the urinal. In the corner, or in the closet."

The frustration in the group is palpable. Rita says, "Jim had a chair he used like a toilet. There was a kind of logic in how he did it. I searched and searched for the source of the odor, the terrible odor. One day, on impulse, I raised the cushion. There was this terrible stain. He had simply raised the cushion as though it were a toilet lid and urinated in the seat of the chair, covering his evidence."

She begins to laugh. "He played with his zipper. Up and down. Up and down. We tried to pin it, lock it, belt it. There was no keeping him from that zipper. They wanted to put him in a jumpsuit at Bright Haven. They were annoyed by his zipper trick. Actually, he was quite unpopular because of it. They implied I should do something about it. I told them I also found it annoying. That was one reason he was there. Because he had behavior problems I couldn't control. He broke everything. He peed everywhere.

"The children were mortified by his behavior. They had ways of covering for him. They never left the room when a friend was visiting, they interrupted when he talked nonsense, and they covered his idiocy with jokes. I remember once my younger son was lying on the floor in front of the TV, and he let out a yell – 'Hey, Mom!' He leaped up and dodged just as Jim started to urinate in front of the television. That happened when I brought him home from Bright Haven for Christmas. About three months before he died."

There is a moment of silence. As children, we believed such a moment signaled the passing of angels overhead.

Bill, the only man in the group, asks softly, "He died?"

"Yes. He was fifty-seven when he died. He had seizures. He was a big man. Six foot five. So tall. Brilliant. A genius. It's really a joke on me. It was his brains, his ability to talk about everything that attracted me to him. I thought, 'Oh, you, you're so smart.' I couldn't resist. What a joke. He turns into this... pathetic creature. So tragic.

"He had top-secret clearance. Three of us in this group were married to engineers with clearance. Can you imagine their brilliant careers at Bright Haven? Staring into space. Space cadets. It's amazing to me we got to the moon. I have to laugh.

"I think of him in his office. He needed a special card to open the door. He sat there for years in his piles of papers. He produced one little book in all that time. This guy he worked with said, 'Jim, I'm amazed you wrote this.' I never knew how he meant this. I stay away from his business associates. I have for years, although I still sometimes talk to their wives.

"For a long time, I watched him. I wondered about him. He was unusual, eccentric, not like other people. His sense of humor, the way he looked at things. I thought it was his brilliance. For the longest time, I was confused. Now I wonder how many Alzheimer's patients were eccentric from the beginning."

I speak for the first time. "My dad was like that. Really odd, bizarre, not like other people." Mother looks engaged rather than shocked. "He was the family genius. And yet, he played a trick on us. I think it took us much longer to catch on than it might have if we hadn't the family mythology of Daddy's eccentricity to sustain our denial, our hope."

"Do you think he was clever at disguising his symptoms?" Rita wants a pattern. I do too.

"It wasn't that he disguised them so much as that he had already established his right to be a nonconformist and an introvert. For years while growing up, I remember believing that Daddy was thinking about important ideas when he was detached or distant. He always carried a slide rule in his pocket. He read. He worked on problems. He designed and executed projects. And nobody expected casual human interaction from him. Not that he never gave it, but when it came, it was an unexpected gift."

"Do you think the early stages of his disease were obscured by his personality?"

I consider the possibility. "Now as I sort through his belongings, I'm puzzled by the numerous elementary math books he has collected. He was acquisitive, always. He bought used books because they were for sale, not because he needed them. But now I'm finding boxes and boxes of books that he might have been using for review. After his bicycle accident, he used to joke that he could always teach trig if he became simpleminded. He expected mental impairment. We all dismissed the evidence he presented to us to support that expectation. We knew he was still so much more intelligent than ordinary people that we really refused to listen to him while he was assessing his own state of mind. Now I worry that we refused him comfort and reassurance."

Rita probes, "And the people at his school probably saw his decline before you would acknowledge it?"

Now I am overcome with a sense of having ignored the most startling and undeniable evidence. I recall how he abandoned his dissertation after I was unable to help with revisions. I felt guilty that I couldn't deal with its mathematical content. I remember conversations and the repeated and refuted anecdotes we all exchanged, and how we clutched at straws of reassurance. I think of the family game of denial. "I can only guess the lengths to which his administrators and fellow teachers must have gone to protect him. He was reassigned, demoted really, relieved of his administrative responsibilities and moved down from gifted classes to remedial classes."

"Yes. That's the way it happens," says Rita. "I think those who worked with Jim knew before I did. I wondered, but I think they knew. They forced him to go to a psychiatrist before I had a chance to. And the psychiatrist knew right away. But Jim wouldn't admit it. He went into a terrible depression. Withdrew. Sank into silence. That was really worse than the weirdness before he knew. And, of course, he didn't tell me. He thought I'd go crazy if I knew. He was right. Everyone goes crazy, and thinks of murder, and suicide."

Her eyes brighten with tears, as her voice softens. "The autopsy showed that his brain had shrunk. It was much smaller than it should have been. He would fall. He was always black and blue and cut. He died from a subdural tumor pressing on his brain."

Maureen has dark eyes and expressive hands that punctuate her speech. "My husband accused me of having an affair. It was the second marriage for both of us. His first wife had been unfaithful, so when things started to go wrong between us, he grasped at the explanation he knew the best and feared the most."

Susan picks up on the subject of sexuality. "We were driving in the car one day, and he turned to me and commented that what he needed was a wife. At first I was defensive, but then I realized his bland eyes were without accusation. He was looking at me as though I were a mere acquaintance. I knew at once that he didn't see me as his wife, that he didn't recall having been my husband or my lover. He was so pathetically incorrect on one level, and so painfully correct on another. He was in need of a wife. He needed absolute comfort and security. He had a need so deep and wide and awful, he could only call it wife."

There is a prolonged silence. No one looks at her face. Each woman in the room looks inward and backward, experiencing that terrible moment of sexual grief as though it had just occurred.

Susan continues, "I go to see him every other day, to feed him his supper. He's glad to see me. He smiles. He's as excited as a child. But, then, he smiles and is excited for anyone.

"Once I went to New York for two weeks, and he was angry with me when I returned. I was so pleased. I was sure his anger proved that he distinguished me from other visitors. But after you lose sexual responsiveness, everything changes. I couldn't sleep in the same room with him after he was sick. I can't tell you what it was like. He was after me all the time. And I tried to be generous and comforting. You know, after verbal communication has deterio-rated, there is still touch. Then once he stopped right in the middle of making love. He had forgotten what we were doing, how to do it, and who I was. I can't tell you how I felt. Like a prostitute. Like a nothing. Finally, I couldn't put myself through it anymore. I told him I was going through the change, and I was just not as inter-ested as I once was. I told him I'd lost interest, that it wasn't his fault. I promised it would be different after I was through the change."

Ruby says, "My husband couldn't be stopped from driving. You couldn't tell by looking at him that there was anything wrong. He got his license, and I thought, 'Okay, drive.' Well, he did. He backed right out of the driveway and right into a car in the driveway across the street. Well, that was that. I just had to let him see he couldn't drive."

"He has a heart blockage," Ruby continues. "I took him to the VA and the treadmill was broken, so they kept him two extra days. I'll know what they want to do when they get the tests back."

Myra, Ruby's daughter, speaks haltingly. "I think we should plan now what to do if they want to perform open-heart surgery."

Ruby's face is placid. "Yes, he's had this heart condition. After he got home from the hospital, he wanted me to sleep with him. He's the sweetest thing. You wouldn't know there was anything wrong to look at him. He's so good with the yard. He rakes the leaves and trims the hedges. He doesn't talk anymore, but he works and helps out."

Myra searches for reassurance from one after another of the group members. "Mother needs to think about what we'll tell the doctor if he wants to operate. We don't have to let him do it. With the other disease, we have to think about the morality of prolonging his life when we know he's losing his mind."

Anne is her ally. "I wouldn't let them touch him if it were my husband. They could damn well let him die. No bypass for him. I would give anything if he would die."

Myra's facial expression reveals that she thinks Anne has gone too far. Her mother picks up the refrain of sweetness – "Oh, I don't want *my* husband to die. I *love* my husband. He's the sweetest man alive."

Anne is adamant. "I pray my husband will die. What's the value of such a life? They're like animals."

"Well, we'll get the test results on Tuesday."

Myra falters, defeated. "And I want us all to talk this over before then. I don't want to permit open-heart surgery."

"I don't know what else the doctor can do for the blockage."

We all know this dialogue by heart. It is repeated in every family of a demented person. The family members regularly change roles – from villain to heroine, from savior to villain. It would be better were he to die. His life is still valuable. His suffering is immoral. He is precious to me. Just the sight of him helps me to remember who he was. When he is gone, we won't even have that. If I were in his place, I would want to die. If I were in his place, I would want you to kill me. If you loved me, you would kill me.

I resist the urge to side with the daughter. It would be so simple if we would all choose sides. Mother has expressed her sense of detachment from those who are not where she is. As in other progressive diseases, the victims align themselves along the spectrum and pass judgment on those who traverse an easier part of the path. Mother cares for Daddy at home, with only the assistance of her teenaged grandson, William. While she admits that his company is her link to sanity, she is somewhat disdainful of those who have regularly scheduled sitters or nurses. She is particularly disgusted with the complaints of those who have placed their victims in care homes. She is praised for prolonging Daddy's functioning by those who have given up caring for their mates at home. It seems that every mate who has placed a victim in a care home believes that they contributed to the progression of the disease. I am reminded of the futile but stubborn attempts of alcoholics' mates to control or cure the disease, and of their inner certainty that they somehow caused it.

Rita addresses me. "And what do you think of what your mother is doing?"

I turn from Rita to Mother. "I tell everyone that I think you're amazing. I don't know anyone with as much courage."

"I don't know if it's courage, or if I'm kind of dumb." The young farm girl inflection takes me by surprise. "Maybe it's just stubbornness. Or maybe it's not being able to decide what to do or when to do it. Maybe my virtue is indecision. People tell me they don't know how I do it, but maybe I do it because I don't know what else to do."

Maureen has been waiting to continue her story. "When I came to the group for the first time, I was desperate, trapped. I'd been married just ten years. We had only three years together before he was diagnosed. I'd been alone for ten years before that. I raised my daughter alone. After she was gone, I was utterly lost. I'd been her mom and felt that I had no separate identity, no idea who I was. Gradually, I just came to terms with myself. I became interested in other people. It was amazing. Suddenly, I could see that some of the women I worked with really were having fun. And I started going places with them in the evening. I really came into my own."

She speaks to Anne with tenderness. "You will, too. When you begin to really *see* the people around you, they'll know it. They will see what you have to offer. You've got to stop thinking of yourself as a wife. You've taken an apartment and you're on your own, but you have this resentment. You can't free yourself from the idea that forty-two years with your husband should entitle you to a reward. You feel cheated."

Anne nods, wiping her eyes. Maureen continues, "But think of me. I had three good years, wonderful years, with this dear man. When I realized he was going to desert me by losing his mind, I felt like life had played a terrible joke on me. I felt like I had been had. I could see right away that his care would be totally in my hands. His children were delighted he was married to someone who could be the caretaker. I couldn't think of leaving him. All I could think of was killing myself. But now, I feel different. Ask these women if I've changed. I can't tell you exactly how it happened, but I've reached a new level of acceptance. I have changed. I can take care of him and I can take care of myself."

For an instant, all the members of the group are transfixed, open, considering the nature of the grace she describes. She whispers, "I don't know where it comes from, but I have this sense of serenity. I know I will discover what I need to come through this. My neighbors are super."

"My neighbor said she was sick and tired of hearing me yell at my husband when the bathroom window was open," says Ruby. "I didn't realize I was shouting when I tried to get him to go to the bathroom. It takes forever. He hardly understands what I tell him. But I didn't know the neighbors heard, or how I must have sounded."

Myra rolls her eyes in response to her mother's tone of voice.

Rita explains, "We all have neighbors who are tired of hearing us shout, who can't stand our complaints. Some of us find these wonderful moments of strength or even wells of endurance. Others of us find ourselves sounding like fishwives, whining and complaining, full of self-pity."

She continues, "I had a call just this morning from a woman who has been to a few meetings, but who claims the support-group concept is not for her. She feels her problems are unique, and that she can't bear the burden of listening to other people's problems. She called me because we've established a one-to-one relationship.

"She said she was calling just because she wanted someone to know what she was about to do. She said she was planning to take a fatal overdose of pills. I asked her who would take care of her husband if she were gone. She said she didn't care. She just didn't want to think about it. I asked her what her children would do without a mother, with only a crazy father. We talked and talked. I knew she wouldn't kill herself, although she needed to discuss the option. She calls every now and then and tells me she's going to drive her car over a cliff. I tell her, 'Nonsense. With your luck, you wouldn't die, you'd only be maimed.'" Everyone smiles in recognition and sympathy. "She's sure I'm right, and has decided to keep on living."

Bill, who until now has been too shy to speak, enters the conversation. "My daughters did what they could for my wife before we had to put her in a home last month. The four of them would take turns spending a day a week with their mother, and we'd have a cleaning woman in one day as well. But she got so bad that she couldn't be alone, and I couldn't stay home from work with her. The neighbors were complaining. We just couldn't keep her home. I couldn't tell how she felt about going to the home, but of course the girls felt bad. And now I can't quite see what's ahead. I just go to work and come home." He veers away from the solemn moment, adding with a wry grin, "I bark at the dog and the dog barks at me."

"Do you think about going out?" asks Rita.

"Well, yes, I have." Bill and his daughter avert their eyes from each other. "This doesn't seem natural. But yet, what could I tell a woman? I'm not really married, but I'm not divorced. I can't see why anyone would be interested in that kind of an arrangement."

"Do you think about divorce?"

"Well, how would that work?"

"In California, you can divorce a mentally incompetent person. You divide the property, just as you would if the person were normal. Or you can arrange to provide for your mate for the rest of his or her life."

"Well, I don't know how the girls would feel about that."

His daughter remains silent.

Rita continues, "Well, of course, a lot of husbands and wives do divorce their mates or date other people. The president of the California chapter was on the Toni Grant Show. He told Toni that he has found a wonderful new way of life. He loves his wife, he provides for her at home with live-in caregivers, and he has affairs. Everyone wins. It really made me uncomfortable. I don't identify with him."

I ask, "How *do* you decide when a marriage is over?" I am prepared to celebrate my parents' fiftieth wedding anniversary, and for my own sake, I want to know that the marriage is over.

"You know early in this disease that you're alone," says Rita. You may perform marital duties, then custodial and caregiving duties, but you know before long that you're as isolated as any widow. There's no one looking after you."

Bill reaches for his daughter's hand, and without looking into her face, says, "And no one outside a marriage, not even a daughter, can know how hard it is to come to terms with that loneliness." He pauses as she begins to cry. "Or what it is to wake up one morning and to know the person you love is as dead as though you'd put her in her grave."

I DREAM that I am climbing over debris in the skeleton of a home I once lived in. I discover that an amateur builder has added on a garage. It is dark and cluttered. At first, I cannot make out the forms of discarded furniture, the heaps of worn clothing. As my eyes adjust to the scarce light, I discover the outline of my father's lifeless body. I am furious with my mother who has left his body unattended. She has not called a doctor, the police, or the mortuary. She has allowed him to die, and has denied the reality of his death.

I awaken to the raw realization of anger so irrational, so unjust, that I walk through the rooms of my dark house waiting for my heartbeat to slow.

I LAND IN CALIFORNIA with a sense of anxiety. As I climb into the van with my luggage, Daddy's eyes take me in. "How are you fixed for money?"

"I'm fine, Daddy. I have money." I kiss his cheek. If he doesn't know me, he makes a familiar association. I am the one who might need money. Whoever I am. I remember the many times he has offered me money, the many instances of his impulsive and dependable generosity. I describe the flight. I was on a huge plane. Ten seats wide. I can't think what they are called.

"Seven forty-seven." Abrupt. Precise. His eyes alert with self-satisfaction.

He is responsive and alert, *there*, for the first twenty minutes of this week-long visit. His attention, his posture, his focus deteriorate over the next six days. By the end of my visit, he has fallen several times. His body is marked by new bruises and abrasions.

His feet do not receive impulses from his brain. He stands in place, doubled over, looking at the feet that do not move when we urge him forward. One knee, and then the other, will move slightly, but he does not move forward. His gait is destroyed. It is hopeless. He cannot approach, let alone climb, the stairs. Mother prepares the Hide-A-Bed for him and puts him down for the night.

Later, she gets him up to use the urinal. She holds it, urging him to cooperate. They stand for a long time, with no result. Finally, they topple over. "Son of a bitch! How much do you think a man can take?"

His anger is new and threatening. He has never before used swear words. There are stories of Alzheimer's victims becoming abusive and threatening. Mother is furious. She talks to him as though he were a disobedient child. "I'm going to take you to the hospital and leave you for three months."

Linda and I leap on her anger, savage with resentment and frustration. "We don't want you to stay with him until you become abusive. You must know when to give up. No one can endure the strain."

She is a passenger on an erratic roller coaster, veering recklessly between poles of solicitude and accusation. She calls him "sweet baby," cooing words of comfort and tenderness, and then she jerks his arms while attempting to pull his rigid body out of a chair. She is the medium between his mute world of phantoms and garbled images and the daily domestic hell to which they are both condemned.

She frightens herself with fantasies of revenge, torture, murder. The radical, ultimate solution to the nightmare seems more attainable than the release she could gain by admitting him to a care home.

*I*T IS NOVEMBER, 1954, a month before John and I plan to marry, *when John calls from Pennsylvania to tell me his father has died. John explains to me that his family has customs I might find difficult to understand. "The coffin is in the parlor," he whispers over the telephone, "and my father must not be left alone before the funeral. You can probably hear the rosary." And what I hear is the hum and murmur of his mother and her mourning sisters, daughters, and nieces.*

When I arrive at his home in Pennyslvania, he whisks me past the parlor, explaining, as I glimpse his dead father, that all the mirrors in the house are covered, all the pictures turned to the wall in keeping with Hungarian Greek-Catholic custom. These symbols remind everyone who passes in the street or who enters the house that normal life has ceased, that grieving and living are separate and distinct. His old aunts — dressed in black, wearing babushkas on their bent heads, singing under their breath to well-worn beads — mourn together as they have all their lives. His mother's widow's weeds are the outward signal that her inward state must be attended to. Although her daughters remind her that navy and dark brown are acceptable substitutes for black, she is unyielding in her determination to "mourn the old country way." While she has confessed that she had wanted to return to Hungary after giving birth to four children, and had felt "trapped" with a husband by whom she was to have thirteen pregnancies, she fiercely mourns his passing and the harshness of her life as one entitled to the sympathy of those around her.

M Y MOTHER'S Alzheimer's support group reminds me of the mourning sisters of John's mother as it gathers to give voice to shared sorrow every first Thursday. The women bind themselves together in anonymity. In their neighborhoods, they are often shunned — modern lepers whose spirits are tainted by the suffering to which they bear witness. If they wore black, if they were veiled in the outward symbol of sorrow, would they be honored, or would they be ignored?

I consider the wife of Job, and, when I realize how vaguely I recall her, I reread the book. She begs Job to "curse God and die." He retorts, "Be silent, foolish woman." No comfort here for a woman who shares and vicariously bears the suffering of her mate. It is Job who is pitied. It is the wife of Job who is silenced and scorned.

A MONG THE LETTERS Nana saved, I find Daddy's letter to the Selective Service. Although he considers himself a pacifist, and would prefer to live in a world in which pacifism were a viable choice, he requests that his classification be changed from that of a conscientious objector. "In light of statements that I made at the time of the registration I can readily see how I came by such a classification. However, my definition of an imperialistic war at that time was hasty and ill chosen, and subsequent events have certainly made it obsolete. My horror of war is as intense as ever. But, the inexorable march of history these past few years calls for a restatement of my position with relationship to the war. My hatred of fascism is and always has been greater than even my hatred of war. Considered with reasoned objectivity, fascism can only lead to war, a degradation of man, and ultimately to the destruction of civilization. I am a believer in democracy, economic as well as political, for therein lies the hope of man for a better world and a lasting peace."

Tommy and I argue.
"It's my turn."
"You had the last turn."
"Mama. He's cheating again."
Daddy's voice is stern. "Hush. Listen."
The announcer's voice seems to come from the orange-lit dial:

"*Bombs... casualties... Japanese... war....*" *The words are pushing my parents together into the only embrace I am to remember from my childhood. Now they are smaller and more frightened than I have ever seen them. Now they are talking, and I know that what we have had— the playground at the school, the field between the house and the trees where we have our hideout, the worn pages in the readers at school, marbles and paper dolls—all these things were part of something invisible, unspoken, called peace.*

We mustn't be afraid. But they are talking, talking, late at night in the living room, and even after they have turned off the lights and gone to bed. I sleep in an iron bed painted white, and although the walls of the room are pink, the moon's reflection on the snow transforms the midnight room to silver. The dolls sleeping beside me with eyes closed become the babies whose houses will be bombed, whose mamas and daddies will be killed.

And Daddy must go to California to find a job in a factory or he will be drafted like my young uncles. We wait for the mail. Mother reads his letters and packs boxes and waits for letters and tells us not to worry. California will be fun. We'll eat oranges and see the ocean. And Mama and Tommy and I are going to drive there all by ourselves. Nana and Grandad are worried about a woman and two small children on the highways alone, but we'll help Mama stay awake, singing "California, here I come, right back where I started from" at the top of our voices.

We are afraid and it is wonderful. The desert is not sand. It has rocks and even trees. And then there is a highway with roses growing on both sides of the road. And miles and miles of orchards. And Mama saying, "I'll just get out of the car and steal myself an orange. There are plenty. Who'd miss one orange? Or even three?" She's like that. Sometimes I am afraid she won't obey the law. Like driving on the wrong side of the road. She likes to drive on the wrong side of the road "when no one's coming, anyway."

Daddy says you must never drive on the wrong side of the road, just as you must never even play with toy guns because even playing with toy guns makes you think war is a way of settling things. And even driving on the wrong side of the road when it's safe might let you forget when it's not and lead to an accident. And there are miles and miles to go.

No, we're not there yet. We can't see Long Beach from here. We'll see towns before we see the ocean and towns before we see Daddy and the housing development. All housing developments have playgrounds and lots of friends for all the kids coming from Kansas and Oklahoma. There'll be plenty of kids to play with who don't talk a bit different and whose daddies don't have to go fight because they have to build planes and ships and tanks to help our boys over there.

"Over there. Send the word. Send the word. That the Yanks are coming, the Yanks are coming . . . "

They teach you how to build ships at the shipyard, so even if you don't know how when you get the job, you have a boss and blueprints and if you have a degree from K.U. and learned how to multiply so you could be an engineer, you can build a ship that won't leak. Daddy is very smart and got straight A's in everything. Except for penmanship, of course. He has the worst handwriting any grownup could have. And English, because he could never think of enough to say because he's so quiet and shy. But he was a whiz at math and science which comes in handy now that we have to fight this awful war and he has to help.

And now we see him. Waving, running down the sidewalk, smiling, smiling. Showing us our apartment. We live in Long Beach, California. We are together in California. We are going to see the ocean. As far as you can see, there is nothing but ocean. And we can take off our shoes and wade in the surf which chases us back and forth, back and forth, whishing, whispering.

SOMETIMES I don't want others to see him, then sometimes I think they should. Why should I have all the pain?" Mother seems to drive faster when she discusses her anger. "It's an epidemic. People need to know the reality of the disease. It's like aging, like death."

We arrive at Bright Haven, a modern California sanitorium, located on a busy street. Mother has explained that it is a locked facility, euphemistically called a "convalescent home," that admits only ambulatory patients. Bonnie and Ruth, members of her support group, have placed their husbands here. While they complain about the conditions at the home, they are both convinced that it provides the best care available in this price range. The director introduces us to an attractive, smiling nurse who will be happy to show us around. Mother explains that she has been here before, but that her daughter needs to see the facility so she can help with "the decision."

No amount of preparation prevents the shock you experience when you leave the world in which the disabled mingle with the able-bodied and enter a world inhabited only by the mentally disabled. I have been responsive to Mother's offer to show me Bright Haven. I want to carry this off with bravado. Still, it is difficult to keep my bearings. I cannot imagine Daddy wandering in these cold corridors with these vacant-eyed strangers. Or perhaps I can imagine him all too readily. He would be so frightened by all these people. Indeed, they are ambulatory. Every resident seems to be wandering aimlessly in the halls. Yet most of the people seem to be oblivious to the presence of the others. They share mutual isolation. They do not seek recognition in the eyes of the strangers they pass. If they speak, they seem to speak to imaginary companions rather than to their fellow residents.

Mother and the nurse talk easily. The nurse is explaining how she met her second husband as we greet Bonnie, who is visiting her husband Fred.

Bonnie gives us a bright, trembling smile. She is formal as she introduces me to Fred, almost as though she expects him to respond. He sits in a chair with an attached plastic tray, staring at the wall behind us, groping for the cookies she continually presses into his hand as she speaks of his improvement.

"Fred is so pleased to be up and around this morning. We've

had a lovely visit. He's enjoying these vanilla wafers, although I probably should make him wait until after lunch to eat them."

"Well, I know he's glad for a special treat," Mother comments.

"I'll bet he'll have an appetite by lunch time," I say, as I realize that we are talking about him in the third person.

The nurse rescues us from our bad manners. "Tell me your name, honey," she implores. "You knew your name just yesterday. Or was it the day before?" She turns to Bonnie. "I know you think I'm making that up, but he did, he told me his name. Plain as anything."

Bonnie's eyes fill. Her smile does not waver. "I believe you. I know Fred remembers his name." She searches Mother's face for reassurance. "And he also remembers my name. He remembers that I am Bonnie and he is Fred. And that we have been married for years and years."

Mother has assured me that Daddy is not nearly as bad as the other residents of Bright Haven. But now that I have seen them, I'm not so sure he would be considered "ambulatory" by the home's standards. As we leave, I voice my concern that he may have deteriorated beyond the point that he could be admitted. If the residents of Bright Haven are unable to walk safely, they are confined to chairs with constraints.

Mother is defiant. "I imagine they would simply strap him into a chair or a bed if he were a resident here. They would not allow him to wander about as I do, knowing that even if he falls, he at least lives in freedom." Defensively, she asks, "What do *you* want for him? Do you want him safely strapped into a chair or tucked into a bed, or do you want him to be able to move about until he is no longer physically able to do so?"

I recall the surprise I felt when my second child, J. D., stood alone at eight months. I was determined that he was too young to stand, that he lacked the judgment to move freely in the house. I attempted to discourage him from standing by arranging toys on the floor, and, finally, by giving him a box of animal crackers. He could not be distracted. He stood again and again, tottering until he fell, and then struggling until he stood, only to fall again. The disease is like a boomerang that sweeps its victims from maturity back through time to a dreadful childhood. Daddy is the determined toddler, standing, falling, then standing again.

I am silenced by how shocked I am by Bright Haven. I realize that Mother is waiting for me to either reassure her, or to stop insisting on this alternative. We play musical chairs with the guilt, each of us unwilling to confront the limits of caring, both of us confused by the dilemmas of responsibility.

"Mother, I know only you can decide when you need to let go. I know it isn't helpful to have the rest of us try to help you decide. I know the guilt is inescapable. But don't believe the women who tell you they think of bringing their husbands home from Bright Haven. They may dream of finding a time warp, of recovering the husband of the past. But by the time a woman has become so exhausted and hopeless that she takes her husband to Bright Haven, she must feel both guilt and relief, both sorrow and freedom."

"Bonnie says she knows Fred would have found some way to have kept her at home if this had happened to her."

"But how can she know that? What is she afraid of? Of knowing the limits of her own devotion, and suspecting that he had the same limits?"

"Well, what is marriage? When does it end? Does it end when your mate no longer knows you?"

"If marriage is commitment, does it end when one person can no longer understand the commitment?"

"Does 'till death do us part' mean only physical death? Or does it mean emotional, social, psychological death?"

Definitions form and disintegrate in the shadow of ambiguity as I shift perspectives. I want my mother and father to prove the reality of the ideal marriage. I want to see that their marriage can survive even the ravages of this disease. But do I want that proof even if my mother is imprisoned and destroyed? What about the wishes of the long-ago father? He would have raged against the sacrifice of one life for another. He would have seen this struggle as a matter of principle, and he would have insisted that the surviving mate had a right to life and freedom. He believed in euthanasia. He believed in cremation. His only hereafter was that of the next generation. But this father is a child who needs security from his hallucinations and nightmares. He is a child who needs his wife to become his mother. He needs to sleep secure in his own bed, lulled by the rising and falling voices of grownups sitting up late in the living room. Grownups ready to ward off bears and monsters.

He needs.

THE NEXT SANITORIUM is California-motel architecture, with many windows overlooking a series of courtyards. Patients who are ambulatory fill the hallways. Some of them respond to us, but most are vacancies. Mother reassures me that "most of these people are much worse than Daddy."

I refuse to go along with her denial, suspecting that she has brought me here to horrify me, and to squelch my constant suggestions that she send Daddy away. "No, Mother, I don't think so. I think Daddy is in a more advanced stage than some of these people."

An old man, bent but bright-eyed, grasps the arms of a passing nurse. She gives him a kiss on the cheek. He turns toward us, smiling and walking taller as he passes, humming under his breath.

Most of the patients sit and stare into space. Those who shuffle about seem to be oblivious to their surroundings, but are often responsive to someone who initiates an exchange.

I have smelled care homes in which the ammonia overpowered the disinfectant, but here, it's a draw. I fight the revulsion I have always felt for these kinds of institutions. The ghosts of Grandpa Ford, Nana, and Grandad flit past and disappear.

"The patients wear clean clothes, but they don't always get their own clothes back from the laundry. Can you tell how many are wearing the clothes of other people?"

I think about the future, my heart sinking. Will he lose his identity here? Will he become a vacancy, not only to himself, but to others who look through him, and to the caregivers whose automatic sweetness and solicitude seem so impersonal?

*I*N THE DREAM, *I am watching the sky. I am surrounded by people who crowd a tiny island. The air is heavy and dark. We know there will be a hurricane. We must all leave quickly. I want to watch and wait. I am not certain the hurricane will really reach the island. The sky is streaked with dark clouds against a navy background. I see hints of lighter blue and pink. Enough good colors to allow me to deny the inevitable storm. Then, suddenly, a cold, harsh wind rises. There are hundreds of people on the dock, and much confusion. There are long, tank-like helicopters coming toward us. People scramble into them. There are sudden ferries against the dock, laden with frantic passengers. I think about climbing a narrow, ribbon-like bridge to reach a hovering helicopter. I am afraid. The wind is so strong now that I imagine the helicopter plunging into air pockets and diving into the water.*

I am on a ferry, near the back, jammed between struggling people who threaten to fall overboard. I move forward, and feel the ferry moving. My panic subsides. One of the boat workers approaches the captain, holding out a black box. The captain opens the box. His face is stricken. I see that the box is filled with dead birds. I shrink back.

He tosses the birds overboard. I do not know where they came from, or how they died.

I ATTEND my second Alzheimer's group meeting with Mother. Beth is a soft-spoken, pretty woman in her early thirties. She attends meetings from time to time with her father, according to Mother. Tonight she has come alone.

"My mother is at home with Daddy. He takes care of her. I try to help. I took her to a baby shower recently because I thought she would enjoy it. But it was impossible to explain. How do you explain presents for a baby not even here? She was terrified someone would ask her a question she couldn't answer. 'How many children did I have?' she asked. She doesn't know that there are four of us, or that I am her child. She wanted to go home before the hostess had even served the dessert. 'My mother doesn't know where I am,' she said. She always says that, although her mother has been dead forty years. I never knew her mother, my grandmother. My mother can't reach me, her forgotten daughter, because she's reaching for her own dead mother."

Susan's husband died on Father's Day. She has returned to the group "to explain the funeral and autopsy arrangements for the benefit of others," she says as though she fears she no longer has a legitimate reason for attending meetings, or as though she is trying to reestablish her own goals for the meetings. "He had an easy death. I knew exactly what to do. I had been making lists, because they told me the end might be near. I reached the brain bank an hour after I was notified. The pathologist removed his brain, but you couldn't tell. His body looked fine in the coffin."

She discusses the "arrangements" with the kind of dreamy detachment one often observes in the bereaved before the dailiness of mourning has overwhelmed them. She reminds us that "when the time comes," we must remember to notify the brain bank immediately, and to have the body chilled until the brain has been removed. Otherwise, the brain tissue will not be in good condition for the tests that must be performed to confirm that the deceased was, indeed, an Alzheimer's victim.

Her directness, her clinical approach to the subject, allows us to satisfy our morbid curiosity.

I ask, "Do they remove the whole brain? Somehow, I thought they would remove only portions of brain tissue to go on microscopic slides."

"It must leave a large, empty space," one woman says.

"Maybe they fill the cavity with some other substance."

"No, they don't. They leave the skull empty."

"You can't tell by looking at the face. They look good," Rita reassures. I recall my first meeting with the group, and her story of her husband's death. It is she who redirects the conversation to the topic of Susan's grieving process.

Susan admits that although she thought she was prepared for and would welcome the death of her husband, she found herself encouraging the doctors to use every possible antibiotic to battle the infection that eventually killed him.

Eva's husband has just returned to the care home from the hospital where she had him transported by ambulance after convincing herself that he had suffered a stroke. She is a woman who has expressed the most matter-of-fact acceptance of the degenerative inevitability of the disease. She now admits with some embarrassment that she "became hysterical," and that she should have known that the increased rigidity of her husband's body was an advanced symptom of the disease, rather than some new insult to his body.

Now she is frightened that her husband will be discharged from the care home because they dismiss patients whom they define as "comatose." She is a political activist in the Alzheimer's and Related Disorders Association. I imagine her with a band of women, carrying her husband on a stretcher, knocking on the door of the White House. Ronald Reagan answers the door, and the women lower the stretcher on the porch before turning to walk away. The women in this fantasy carry no banners. They wear no slogans on their T-shirts. Yet their anger centers their lives in protest.

The group members have moved to a discussion of the governmental rules and regulations that restrict care and assistance to Alzheimer's victims. A man who asserts that his wife was first diagnosed with "multiple infarcts" before Alzheimer's disease is advised to "stick with the 'multiple infarcts' diagnosis" so that she will be qualified for treatment rather than custodial care. If the diagnosis qualifies her for treatment, she may be eligible to collect insurance benefits for her hospitalization. Custodial care is disqualified from reimbursement because it is considered to be more beneficial to the caregiver than to the victim of the disease. A newcomer to this group's meeting is outraged by this information.

In a sense, each meeting is a microcosm of the disease. The group members do not conform to the orderly process of the Kübler-Ross stages of grief. During the course of the evening, each woman, in recounting her story, in reporting her week, personifies denial, anger, bargaining, depression, *and* acceptance. And within the hull of each of these emotions there is a kernel of guilt.

Sandra has grown thinner and thinner since her husband's death. She has continued to come to meetings to get help with her failure to come out of the grief process. "He is dead a year, and I feel guiltier now than I did when he was alive. You forget the unbearable aspects of the disease. But not how terrible you were. If I'd known he would only live a year after being placed in the home, I might have been able to endure and to keep him at home. But now I can't imagine how I could have done such a terrible thing to such a dear person. How could I have put him in that awful place when he was so sick, so close to death? I think about it all the time. He was such a wonderful person, and yet I sent him to a care home."

Inevitably, the widow exhumes the guilt she hoped to bury with her husband. She cannot assure Mother and these women who have yet to bury their mates that they will be free from guilt after their husbands die.

DADDY STANDS in the kitchen, staring at the floor as if it were a moving tide. He puts his foot out as the to test the water.

He is startled by the television, as though by an intruder. His eyes glide from the screen to my face and I know by his look of revulsion that he is seeing me as a monster.

He seems to be watching scampering, invisible animals darting about the room. He tries to raise his feet as if he's trying to avoid them. He does not cry out, as he would have a year ago when he reported such apparitions.

I recall his recitation of nonsense syllables one morning as he shuffled in place in the kitchen.

"What's wrong, Dad?"

"There were a series of four bomb explosions."

"Is that what you heard?"

"Didn't you hear them? There were four explosions. There were four pressure bombs that went off."

His eyes demand response. Then he shrugs and his eyes become vacant. I wonder if paranoia is the realization that others ignore the clear and present danger that you know will consume you.

During Linda's Christmas visit, he insisted that she call the Highway Patrol. "The campers are lost in the blizzard. They will be frozen to death by morning. You must call now."

"What campers, Daddy?"

"There is no point in asking questions. Do as I say."

"But we're in California, Daddy. There is no blizzard. There are no campers."

"Listen to me. Do as I say."

She steps across the boundary between their worlds. "The Highway Patrol just called, Daddy. They have found the campers. They've been rescued. They're all safe."

He smiles with relief. For once, his body is not clenched as she tries to embrace him. He does not turn his cheek away as she kisses him. Perhaps it is more healing to yield to his view of the world rather than to insist that he remain in our world.

I TURN THE PAGES of family albums, trying to retrieve the past. One page of the album has a series of photographs in which I befriend a baby cottontail rabbit, learn to love him, release him in the freedom of the woods, and mourn his loss. The last photograph in the series shows a bedraggled and tearful six-year-old.

The caption, in Daddy's handwriting but my words, reads, "If he's happy, I'm happy."

WASN'T IT NICE of Carol to come for our anniversary?" "I should say so." Is this the last sentence I will hear him utter? This visit has brought me to a new resolve. I no longer find myself wanting to coax him into conversation. Now it seems he needs every shred of concentration to remain upright if he is standing, or to move his hands from his plate to his mouth if he is eating.

He requires instructions for moving his feet if he is walking. Mother often stands behind him and pushes him forward. Too briskly, I think. She is exasperated when he stands too long in one place, his knees bending slightly with the misfired impulses which no longer result in steps. He makes nearly disastrous errors on the stairs, now facing the railing and grasping it with both hands, descending until one foot stands on the other, his legs crossed, stuck. One of us bends over beside him, trying to lift the foot he must free to move. When he approaches the stairs correctly, hand on rail, he barely succeeds in placing his toes on the very edge of the tread, so the person behind him waits for him to topple backward. He lifts himself out of a chair with such difficulty that it is agony to watch. He throws himself backward to seat himself, nearly missing the seat and crashing into the arm. To watch him move is to foresee disaster with every motion. I think of people with cerebral palsy, and wonder if we should buy him a helmet for his protection.

He has become a night wanderer. He gets up and partially disrobes, then stands immobile in the hall, having forgotten his destination. Linda awakens Mother when she finds him half-naked and shivering at the top of the stairs. When he falls back on his bed, he is unable to cover himself. Yet the house is kept as cold as it was in the early days of their shared concern with energy conservation.

THERE IS SOMETHING so feisty and ornery in Mother that I am amazed. She reports, her eyes crinkling with pleasure, "He was talking about me in the third person, as though he did not recognize me. I decided to get him to gossip, so I asked him, 'What do you think of Fern? Is she a dictator? Is she too bossy for words?' He didn't miss a beat. He said, 'Oh, no. I love her.' I thought, 'He's still too smart for me. I can't trick him. He knows he's at my mercy.'"

She takes pleasure in his accomplishments as though he were a child growing brighter with each passing day.

"He could spell *Massachusetts*. When I asked him to spell some words, he could spell them all."

Hope flickers in my mind: Is it possible that he could improve?

AFTER RETURNING HOME from a visit, I sometimes feel surprisingly detached. I think, "Why, I have accepted this. I feel calm. I'm not in pain." I am relieved to be so far from my parents' painful existence. Then, after being home for a few hours, I try to recall his image and his last words. I recall Mother asking, "Leonard, wasn't it nice of Carol to come for our anniversary?"

And his response, lyrical with the rhythm of courtesy," Why, I should say so." The memory of this single instance when he seemed to still be himself is somehow comforting to me even though it became clear to me during the remainder of the visit that he no longer recognized me.

I am *not* calm. I have *not* come to accept his ravaged condition. For weeks following my departure from him, I fight the impulse to telephone at hourly intervals. It is as though he is in intensive care, having barely survived a terrible accident. I need to be there, by his side. I am besieged by lucid dreaming, awakening with his image vivid, demanding.

A T MY PARENTS' HOUSE, I'm angered by open cupboard doors, frayed furniture, and cracked teacups. I hate the absence of simple comforts and decencies. I want to make order, but I try to resist venting the anger I feel. I try to stop making suggestions and giving advice to Mother. After all, I have never been a conscientious housekeeper. Yet I want her to have a garage sale. I want to be rid of all the books that won't ever again be read, and all the camping equipment that won't ever again be loaded into the van. The typewriters, adding machines, cameras, bicycles, hammers, saws, tree-trimmers—all the symbols of Daddy's work and leisure, all the symbols of his hobbies and interests–all these things hurt. I want them gone. I want order. Emptiness. Closure.

I PERSUADE TOM to come to Mother's house to help restore order. We walk around the neighborhood, and I find myself breathless from my anger and from the exertion of the walk. Tom is detached and philosophical. He lives in a calm, beautiful world of his own making and permits our parents their own disorder.

"I've reconciled to the fact that Mother won't make any decisions. There will have to be a crisis. Then we'll have to be ready to take over. She won't get rid of the trailers, the camping equipment, the office equipment, or anything." He adds wryly, "I'm surprised you returned, knowing she hadn't held the garage sale after your cleaning spree of last summer."

"What is more surprising than my return is my silence." He knows that I usually drive a hard bargain with others. Who knows better than a younger brother the control needs and harsh judgment of an older sister? Who has a more auspicious position than he for developing patience and philosophical detachment?

I promise myself I will simplify my life. If I long for order, it is my task to make it for myself rather than imposing it upon others.

How many other mothers and daughters divide themselves over style? The choices of quality, the symbols of value? She won't part with the trampoline in the backyard. Who knows what dear memory it evokes for her? When I see the faded canvas and the rusting metal frame, I mentally haul it off and plant flowers in its stead.

I can't untangle the ambivalence I feel for this tough little white-haired seventy-year-old woman who drives her van in L.A. traffic as though she was shooting the rapids with the wind at her back. I want her to buy a practical, compact car, one more appropriate for transporting an invalid. Yet she clings to all the trappings of their adventurous days. She clings to her faded jeans and hiking boots just as she clings to that pioneer aspect of herself which sees me as too cautious, too domesticated.

She often appears to be so young, so optimistic, so undaunted, that I find myself becoming mother to her child.

I see our identities as flecks of colored glass, falling into exotic, intricate patterns that shift with the kaleidoscopic whirl of the moment. One moment she seems broken, victim of a vicious fate. The next moment she seems as indestructible as a mother goddess with her hands in the mud of creation. Then she seems as flippant as a girl, dancing in a high-school rendition of "Tiptoe through the Tulips."

*S*OMETIMES HE'S NOT NICE *to my dolls. Sometimes he tosses them about as though they had no feelings. He doesn't remember their names. Raggedy Ann. Paulette. Sandra. Susan. Jennifer. I haven't enough beds for all of my children. If I put some of them down on the sofa for a nap, he may sit on them, without looking. He never allows me to take them all on a trip to the beach or to Long Beach. I must choose which two may go, and then remember who I must leave at home next time. I try to tell them why he is so mean to them. They try to understand how he is. Still, those who are left at home are sorry, even when I bring them Cracker Jack prizes or ticket stubs from the roller coaster on the Pike.*

I AM A LITERATURE MAJOR who longs for plot and structure. I habitually try to mold my life experiences into a literary model. I would like to see all suffering as heroic. I want Daddy to become a hero who journeys through the valleys of despair only to be transformed by revelations at the heart of danger.

Families touched by Alzheimer's disease are desperate for sequence. When we meet, we can hardly listen to the other person's trials, we are so eager to testify to the collapse of order in the life of the person now at the center of our family. Whether the victim is ignored or attended to, he is inevitably the focus of attention. We wear his illness as widows once wore weeds, to announce the presence of death in all life.

And we are shunned as we clutch at the attention of indifferent passersby, announcing to their deaf ears, "My father-in-law was a kind man, a gentle man, and we knew, when he chased his wife of sixty years with a butcher knife, that he had to be sent to a home."

Or, "She was a model of patience until he cut the bedsheets into shreds, and she knew then that he was beyond her."

"He started yelling obscenities at her, and then, one day, he twisted her arm. Then she knew she was looking into the face of a stranger, an enemy, not the man she had loved since she was a girl."

And we recite our grievances against those with whom we share our pain. We discover ourselves telling our co-workers and neighbors the intimate details of family betrayals, as though determined to bring them to judgment. "My mother has always been angry with my father for controlling the finances and the decision-making. Now when I see the bruises on his arms, I wonder if he has fallen or if she has been abusive."

And, "Mother is furious with the boys. Their dad doesn't recognize them anymore, but she wants them to visit him at the care home to show respect. You'd think they would do so out of respect for her, but they won't. They stay away from him, and eventually they will stay away from her. She is no comfort to them, and they are losing a father. But she feels bitter and accuses them of neglect. They hear themselves condemned and become neglectful."

"When she was a baby, her mother nursed her and comforted her, and treated her like a princess. Now that Mother is ill, do you think she can bring herself to so much as touch that crippled old body? She won't give her any personal care. Won't brush her teeth, or shampoo her hair or bathe her. She says professional nurses are trained to do such things. She always thought she was too good to work like the rest of us."

Alzheimer's disease is a family disease. It is like cancer or alcoholism or any degenerative disease because it reminds us all of our mortality and of the temporal nature of family roles. The family is a system that delicately balances rights and responsibilities. Few of us are prepared to relinquish roles with grace and dignity. The disease is a mirror from which we turn away.

We idealize the victim's once healthy persona and shrink from the pathetic hull we see him becoming. All of us bear our secret guilt. We are afflicted with survivors' guilt before and after the physical death occurs. We see ourselves condemned in the disintegration of the other and in the involuntary flinching of those who cannot look at the victim. We are twice threatened with the limits of our physical and spiritual possibilities.

And always we are thwarted by the absence of plot. As the victim moves through a regressive tunnel into a past from which we are excluded, we find ourselves abandoned and bereft, contemplating the irrational. We want design in this chaos. We wish to be ennobled by the suffering of the other, so that we might close our ears to the sound of his whimpering in the night.

I DRAW A LINE down the center of the bed, telling Tommy yet again to stay on his side. I watch the dark shapes within the closet move for a few seconds before closing my eyes against the possibility of the prowler who lurks in the closet every night at bedtime. From the living room there is the sound of the purring radio, the fluttering pages of the newspaper as Mother reads aloud to Daddy.

"You sing first."

"I sang first last night."

He gives in, singing in a voice that rises only slightly above a whisper.

> Over there. Over there.
> Send the word. Send the word.
> That the Yanks are coming.
> The Yanks are coming.
> And it won't be over
> Till it's over over there.

I sing to Tommy, imagining myself grown, encircled in the arms of a screen-sized man who resembles Johnny Thomas.

> There'll be blue birds over
> The white cliffs of Dover
> Tomorrow, just you wait and see.

The door opens suddenly. "You kids go to sleep. It's past your bed-time." Mother's voice is stern.

We play possum. I feel the quiver of Tommy's stifled giggles as the door closes. We snuggle into a shivering knot of suppressed laughter.

"We'd better just tap the tune," I whisper.

We move into the next round of the bedtime game. I tap out a tune on his back. He guesses "Sentimental Journey" after only a few bars. I must remember not to do that one again. He guesses it too easily.

I turn away from him so he can tap on my back. He, too, repeats his fa-vorite songs.

> Anchors aweigh, my boys.
> Anchors aweigh.
> Farewell to college joys.
> We sail at break of day, day, day, day.

I drowse for a moment before I guess. "Anchors Aweigh."

"You always get that one. Let me do another." He forgets to whisper.

"You'd better hope I don't come in there." Daddy's voice has that 'this is the last time I'm warning you' tone. We hold our breath. I count to my-self until the hum of Mother's voice assures me that he has been dis-tracted.

Tommy taps his tune on my back, cheating by tapping faster than the tempo of the tune. I give up. He turns away from me, facing the wall. I move close, taking in his Ivory soap smell, feeling the soft soles of his smaller feet on the tops of my feet. We are spoons. We are two snug bugs in a rug.

*T*OMMY IS THE FIRST ONE *to spot the truck as we round the corner. The sign on the door of the truck reads "Sears, Roebuck and Company." The two delivery men carry a huge box between them. We race into the house to see shiny maple bed frames assembled in the tiny den.*

Mother beams. "It's your new bunk beds, Tommy. You're a big boy. Daddy says you're too big to sleep with Carol. Daddy says . . . "

At dinner, I ask, "Could we wait? How would it be if he just sleeps with me one more night?"

Daddy's eyes cool to gray. His voice is firm. "Boys and girls share a room only when they are children. It won't be long before you are grown. Soon, you'll go through puberty." The new word bristles with dangerous significance. I am eager to leave the table.

He addresses Mother as though I have been excused. His jaw flexes. He looks past me at Mother. "I told you it was time." He rises and stalks out of the room without excusing himself. He mutters to himself, "Or past time."

M Y SISTER LINDA and her son William wrestle as she tries to force him onto her lap to once more be her baby. Proud of his newly acquired height, he holds her wrists above her head, taunting her with his recognition of her helplessness, her submission to his sudden stature. She laughs until the tears come. Watching, I recall the mingling of pride and sorrow when I knew my baby Jeff had become a man.

The moment of William's passage becomes a freeze-frame as we hear Daddy crashing down the stairs, moaning and grunting as his body strikes each step. When we reach him, he is curled into a tight fist at the foot of the stairs. He is silent, staring at the wall.

Mother croons words of comfort, to us as much as to him. "There, there, sweetie. You're all right. Now. Now. Don't you worry. You're going to be fine. Just take a minute to get your bearing. Here, honey, does this hurt? Feel your arms. Are they okay? Let me feel your forehead. I don't think you've cracked your skull."

His body is rigid. William tries without success to move Daddy's legs, then his arms. Finally, Mother moves a chair close to him, and waits for him to grasp the leg of the chair. After doing so, he manages to push himself up on his hands and knees, and he climbs to his feet, using the chair to stabilize himself.

I watch with the sense of detachment that comes and goes. I feel myself move beyond empathy into a quiet, troubled place.

In the middle of the night, I hear him cry out. Linda gets up to comfort him. I go back to sleep. I sleep without dreaming.

NOW THAT HIS SENSE of logic is gone," Linda reflects "he can no longer analyze or impose order on others, or on the world. Perhaps he is reduced to his mystical essence. Perhaps he is in a purer, trancelike state. I want to think his mind has turned to spirit. His perception has turned to light."

"I would like that, too. Purity. Simplicity. Not bereft of language, but beyond language."

But the image of his bent and diminished body, tilting and stiffened, naked below the waist, his eyes locked into a tunnel of horror, is there. And the sound of the caged animal within him, moaning. The primal chorus heard in the halls of care homes throughout the world echoes in our minds. Daddy makes a sound common to Alzheimer's victims: "Kitty, kitty, kitty, kitty."

I STAND BEHIND HIM, my arms locked around his waist. He leans toward the stairs, looking intently at a phantom lurking on the bottom stair.

"Come sit down. Come with me, Daddy, dear. Daddyboy."

I feel his will move forward, downward to the space at the bottom of the stairs. His feet, however, are stuck in place. He is mute, focused. Fifteen minutes pass. He is beyond my coaxing. I turn him toward the living room, thinking he may follow if I precede him. As I turn my back, glancing over my shoulder, he begins to teeter wildly, unable to gain balance or break his fall. He strikes his head on the corner of the stairwell, lies like a stick at my feet.

His eyes are unblinking. He is silent. He doesn't wince or moan. I don't move for a long time. Then, I place a pillow under his head, determined to wait for Mother to help me pull him to his feet. When she returns from an errand, she is calm and patient, instructing him so that he can help her get him to his feet.

We inspect the welts under his shirt and on his head. These welts will bloom into tomorrow's bruises.

No mystical purity here. I recoil from my helplessness, my failure to protect this pitiful, wounded, dying creature.

*S*HE'S A BATTLE-AX. *She wears a navy crepe dress with a Kate Smith neckline over which her goiter swells as do her ankles above the brown lace-up oxfords with stacked heels. Her wispy hair unties itself from the small tight knot at the nape of her neck.*

She's put my name on the after-school list for drawing Mopsy instead of listening to her telling us what she already told us yesterday about the rainfall in the Amazon. She expects us to remember what grows there. Not who lives there. There are no people in geography. There are cultures and tribes, but no people. There are numbers of bushels of grain. There are ranges of degrees of Fahrenheit or Centigrade per season. Numbers to memorize. Charts to study. She wants us to memorize numbers forever. I want to wait until the day before the test, so I will know them as briefly as possible before forgetting them, as I intentionally do when a test is behind me. If I knew all the facts she knows, I would be like her. I would get a goiter and fat ankles, and steely gray eyes that see through the raised desktops of students who are minding their own business.

Mopsy has short, curly dark hair, huge eyelashes, and a turned-up nose over pouty lips. The cartoonist mostly draws her profile, which I can do exactly. From the side view, you would swear I was the cartoonist. I draw her over and over, for hours. She has high, round breasts over a wasp waist and swelling hips which flow into long, slender legs.

I always draw her in a bathing suit like the ones Jackie and I are going to have my mother make for us as soon as I get them. The bathing suit is white broadcloth, two-pieced, with the halter gathered over them and tied in the middle, and the bottom has gathers in the front and laces up the sides, so skin shows through the laces. Jackie has had them since the fourth grade. She slouches because she got them early, like I slouch because I'm getting them too late, if ever.

Daddy watches me all the time, not smiling and ordering me to "stand up straight." I hate it when he says that. He's always talking about me to Mother, saying, "Now, Fern, it's time you had a talk with her."

When I get them, I'm going to wear my white Mopsy bathing suit to the beach every day. I will tape the initials "L. D." on the backs of my thighs, and Jackie will tape the initials "J. T." on the back of her thighs, one letter on each leg. Then, we're going to bake. Our suntans will show off our boyfriends' initials. At home, I'll wear jeans so they won't know. It's none of their business anyway. I like to wear jeans rolled up, huaraches, and one of Daddy's old shirts when Jackie and I go to the lot to play football with Louie and Johnny and the gang.

At first I liked Johnny, but then we decided we would draw names for which one of us liked which one of them. This was before they knew we liked them. Now, Louie knows I like him. Jackie told Johnny, and he told Louie. Somehow, Pinky and Patsy Postal found out. Patsy's freckles will surely have all run together by the end of the summer. I don't know what she'll do. And as for her other problems, I'll probably get them before she does, if ever.

Daddy told Mother that they were "going to have to have a curfew," and "talk to Carol about some other things" while they were at it. So, she sat me down and told me in this worried voice, not even looking me in the eye, "Leonard wants me to have a little talk with you, Carol. He says it's time for you to know about some things that will be happening. And he says you're not to play football with the boys anymore. You're much too big to be tackled by those big boys. Isn't that Louie in the eighth grade? Well, at your age, you should stop having that much physical contact with big boys. Soon you'll understand why it's important . . . "

I could have died. Then, she gave me this pamphlet about sanitary napkins, and then a little flat bra for someone who didn't need one. She said Daddy noticed the cotton of his shirts was too thin for me to wear without an undershirt, and she just happened to have this "brassiere," and she thought it would fit me. I could have died. Daddy looks at my chest. He thinks I'm getting them. Or he's worried that I won't get them. He thinks I'm going to get a period. He'll know when I wear a sanitary napkin. Or he'll ask her and she'll tell him. I could die.

Miss Humbert thinks she can make me stay after school, but she has no right to ruin my plans. Jackie and I are going to Long Beach on the bus. We're going to shop at Buffum's Department Store, and then we're going to have a tuna salad sandwich on white toast and a chocolate malt, and then we'll take the bus home along Ocean Boulevard. We know the schedule and the stops, and we only have to transfer once. We'll talk about Louie and Johnny and plan my staying over at her house on Saturday.

We sleep together in her three-quarter-sized bed on her filthy sheets in her messy room. She picks her clothes up right off the floor to get dressed. She never hangs her clothes in the closet or takes anything, even clean underwear, out of her drawers. I love her room. It smells so . . . cozy. I guess it's cozy. She has a dressing table with a flowered chintz skirt to match her bed's skirt. She has cut-out pictures all over the walls. She has a picture of Alan Ladd over her bed on the ceiling. On the ceiling!

Her parents run a restaurant. They both smoke. They're never home. They call her every day after school to check on her. When we go to her restaurant, we can order anything we want, but there is never any food in her house. Sometimes, when I stay over, I offer to make us French toast at my house. That's my specialty, French toast. I make my own syrup with white and brown sugar and water and a dash of maple flavoring.

Miss Humbert is glaring at me. She marches down the aisle and grabs my drawing of Mopsy and holds it up before the class.

"You'll be interested to see what Carol is doing while we are learning about the world around us," she snarls. And, as everyone laughs, she

adds, "And why she is not only going to stay after school today, but every day this week."

The bell rings as if to punctuate her sentence. Before I know what I am doing, I am moving, moving, and am outside the school building. I see Jackie waiting by the corner of the building.

"Hi, kid," she says, as we hurry toward the bus stop.

"I'm afraid we'll miss our bus," I pant, as we break into a run.

Do I hear Miss Humbert shouting at me, or is it only the rush of blood pounding in my ears, as we run, faster and faster?

I AM FATIGUED from my trip. Post-stress syndrome is a useful concept. I rise to the occasion when I visit them. I spend days in rehearsal, and disguise the shock I experience when I first see him. Regardless of how well I think I have come to terms with the degeneration, I still remember him young and well, and find the way he looks now distressing. Mother must find my cheerfulness annoying.

Back home, I try to adjust to the tempo of my work, and to the magnitude of students' problems, but I am vulnerable to unexpected tears. The image of his bent, immobile body intrudes on the moment.

When I am with him, I know we are strangers. When I am home again, I imagine that he knew me. I imagine that he recognized me even though he didn't seem to at the time. I mull over the few seconds during the entire visit when he seemed so much himself. I cannot release him. The person he was. The giant. The all-knowing, all-giving, all-being, all-meaning other. I still believe that man is somewhere. In how many cells? What happens to the cells that held his essence? When do we celebrate the life of that essential being?

I imagine a fall. He breaks his hip and dies quickly, avoiding the more predictable death from starvation or strangulation. Mother has told me that when he cries, he is unable to tell her why he is crying. I rehearse an imagined death for him without tears.

NANA AND GRANDAD cannot grasp the irreversible nature of their eldest son's disease. I visit them in the re-tirement home where they have lived since Nana's stroke.

Grandad is a fixer, a problem-solver, a patriarch whose word has been law for ninety years. He was a car dealer whose retire-ment after the age of eighty-eight has been devoted to honing his ability to bargain with the toughest customer of all. He thinks he can barter with God. He has subscribed to an offer advertised by Oral Roberts to "expect a miracle," making regular payments of eighty-eight dollars and eighty-eight cents for the restoration of movement in Nana's right arm and right leg.

"I want you to write to Tommy to ask him to pray for Leonard."

"Leonard has a progressive, degenerative disease of the brain, Grandad." I have made a decision that this old man will die know-ing who I am. I strive to break the lifelong family-sanctioned habit of telling him only what he wants to hear. "Prayer may not be the answer." I never stand up to him without inwardly quaking.

"Now, you don't know until you try. Tom would try for a mir-acle."

I wonder if he feels that he has been asking for too much lately. Does he think he's being personally punished because Nana hasn't gotten any better? Although he swore he saw her toe move months ago, he has not alluded to additional signs of progress. Al-though I discount his religious faith, I find his tenacity comfort-ing.

"If Leonard had been a churchgoer . . . "

"If Leonard had been a churchgoer, then what?" My sympathy becomes defiance.

"Then . . . "

"Then this might not have happened? He might not have become ill?"

"Well, maybe not... "

"Then you think God punished him for his atheism by giving him a brain disease?"

"Well... "

"Have you ever known a better man than my father?" I realize that my loyalty on this issue has prevented my saying "your son."

"I can't say as I have... "

"Was he a good son, a good husband, a good father, a good worker? Was he a fair person who did what was moral in every action he ever took?"

"Yes, I believe so."

"Then, being that kind of a man, if he now finds himself the victim of this kind of curse, what can you say about God, Grandad?"

Daddy must have confronted his father in this way when he was a teenager. I am relentless, without pity for his aged fragility. "Isn't a god who would do this to such a good man a monster?"

He is as resilient as he is tough. "Well, maybe it's like you say. A physical disease."

MOST OF OUR SATURDAY CONVERSATIONS are less urgent at the outset than today's. Mother's voice is hollow as her despondency surfaces. She whispers into the receiver, and I picture him sitting on the kitchen sofa, perhaps with a look of confusion evoked by the ringing telephone, as though he himself expected a call.

"I was cranky with Leonard. He wet his pants and I was cross. I couldn't help it. I was tired, and he had been wearing clean clothes. I scolded him."

There is a long silence, then I hear the intake of her breath.

"He cried. He told me he tries so hard. I was so sorry. I make up my mind I'll never be cross, and then I lose my temper. He doesn't have accidents for a while, and then he does."

"Oh, Mother. Oh, dear . . . "

"And it's just too much for one person."

"Of course it is," I say soothingly while waiting for the surge of anger, sharp as pain, to subside.

She continues in a confessional vein. "My friend Jean called and told me about a trip she was planning with her husband. She sounded so happy. I said, 'Well, I'm not going anywhere. I'm just going to see if I can keep from losing my mind. I don't know why I don't lose my mind. I just don't.' Then I said goodbye and hung up. Jean probably thought I was going to kill myself. She called me when she got back from her trip. I guess she wasn't as mad at my outburst as I thought she might be."

I hesitate, wary.

"Well, don't I have a right to feel that way? I was just mad that she was happy and I was stuck. I think I have a right to feel that way."

I falter, knowing that any response to the rage behind that question will entrap us both.

The conversation ends with an evasive ploy. I brag that I have harvested twenty-six strawberries. The smallest strawberries I have ever seen, but twenty-six of them.

I GIVE MY ANGER a week to simmer, then I know I must call her back. I am prepared to confront her negativity, her projection of blame onto friends. I think of my friend Sharon, whose mother has Alzheimer's, calling her parents' home "the house of the living dead." I know that no amount of looking on the bright side or feigning good cheer can assuage the horror a casual visitor, not to mention a friend, must feel at Daddy's gradual death. While his body dies slowly, Mother's vibrant spirit seems to die quickly, so I miss both of the parents I once knew.

She tells me that her sister Esther and her husband are planning a trip to Europe and that they have invited her to join them.

"Then you must go."

"I was afraid to tell you. I knew you would make me go."

"You're right. I insist that you go. If you had a job other than caregiving, you would have a paid vacation. You would never hire a person to care for Daddy and refuse them a two-week vacation. If you consider how much you've saved by taking care of him yourself, even if you calculate costs at minimum wage, you've earned a trip."

I have struck a nerve. "Well, actually much more than this trip," she hesitates, mentally calculating. "When I think what I would have to pay for a person to work one shift a day, and I do three . . . "

"Exactly. And I called to tell you how frightened I was by our conversation last week. You treated your friend Jean as though you were making reasonable demands on her concern and friendship. But you were being crazy. When you hate and envy the pleasure of your friends, you're through. You were blaming her for her good fortune, as though you wished her husband were ill. As though the score between you could be evened. I've been there. I've been in a state where I envied the good fortune of others. It's the ultimate mental illness."

Do I hear her crying on the other end of the line? I'm not sure, but I can't stop. "You're clinically depressed," I say. "You sleep too much. You have no energy. Your interests and relationships are narrowing. You have nothing to look forward to. You do not feel much for other people. Your emotions are flattened. You have every symptom of depression I know. You have every symptom of depression I have ever had. And, even though you may not acknowledge my experience, I am an expert. You're flirting with an extremely dangerous condition. You seem to assume that you can care for Daddy indefinitely. Tom says you will care for him until there is a crisis, that you'll break under the strain. And despite the fact that you seem to be indestructible, I can imagine that you could break and never ever put yourself back together again."

Now I am certain she is crying. I don't care if she hears my tears. I pant with the effort of facing truths I had not known until I heard them from my own lips.

M OTHER IS IN THE TINY KITCHEN of our Seal Beach house, leaning against the edge of the sink, timing a contraction with the clock she has brought from her bedroom to watch while she cans peaches. She has bought the peaches from the fruit and vegetable vendor because they are beautiful, and because she thinks she will have time to can them all before the baby comes... if she hurries. How sensory is vivid memory. The house is fragrant with the steam of the peaches boiling in syrup. Mother wears a long robe of dusty rose and white polka-dotted silk. Above the deeply ruffled neckline, her face glows with the mystery of anticipation. Her eyes are luminous.

Daddy watches her every move as she arranges the hot, sterile jars on the back of the stove, as she spoons the hot peaches into the jars, and as she fishes the steaming lids from the caldron of water. His voice is calm and restrained. Only the twitching of the muscle beneath his earlobe betrays his controlled anger. She is a woman who won't be hurried. He is a man who hates to be late.

This is the first time she has had to go to a hospital to have a baby. She does not want to spend more than one extra minute in the hospital. He thinks ahead to traffic, to the possibility of an emergency, to his enforced passivity. He packs her bag according to the instructions she calls to him as she "puts up" the last of the peaches.

While we wait for the news, Tommy and Aunt Everta and I sit on a blanket spread out on the grass in the front yard. We have left the front door open so we will hear the telephone ring when Daddy calls, and so we can hear the news bulletins on the radio.

He calls to tell us we have a baby sister. I have always known this would be the happiest day of my life. I run up and down the street, shouting the news to my friends, and to all the neighbors. Tommy finds this display very embarrassing. He has said all along that if this baby is a girl, we can send it back.

When Daddy returns, he looks haggard rather than ecstatic. He explains that "the baby came much too fast, but... seems fine." Then he makes a characteristic leap from the personal to the historical level of experience. "We must not be duped by the press into believing that the United States has won the war." He expresses his deep sorrow that we are to grow up in a world in which it is possible to split the atom.

MOTHER AND I talk again about the European trip she is reluctant to take. After spending an angry afternoon and a restless night, I call her back. I insist that she take the trip. I confront her about her negativity, telling her she is sicker than he is, and that her mental health depends upon having time away, time to rest and gain perspective.

She tells me, "Just having his body is something. He's still partly here, even though he's stiff and rigid. I got in bed with him last night, just to be near him. I miss touching. It's so lonely to never have touching, and to have him here, but not here. He's so quiet. Now, when he talks, he whispers. And he can't express himself. Yesterday, he was trying to tell me something, and he couldn't find the words. He started to cry. I tried to comfort him, but he kept crying. I put my arms around him and told him I thought he had done so well and tried so hard. And, that he had always been a wonderful person. I couldn't tell if he understood, but I wanted him to know."

"If one woman were to tell the truth about her life, the world would split open," wrote Muriel Rukeyser. Such is the truth my mother tells, Saturday after Saturday. I spend the week building a wall of reason around my feelings, only to have it knocked down in an instant by her unbearable revelations. I want her to think of having a European tour so I will be free of the thought of her curling beside his rigid body, looking into his absent eyes.

"He comes into my room wearing jeans and the jacket to his silk suit," Mother continues. "He knows it is morning, and he worries that he'll be late, as though he thinks he still has to go to work. And I realize, he's still trying. There's something in him that is fighting this. And there's part of him that is still *him*."

I am sad and angry after we talk. Jana and Jeff tell gross-out jokes at the dinner table, and even though I laugh, I am brooding. Mother has become the plague carrier, and I resent her for this. And because of my resentment, I come to resemble her. I have tried to manipulate the situation so that a trip can give her respite. She has focused my attention on Daddy and his tenacious spirit.

How weary she must be with my lectures, my advice, my harshness. When she tells me about climbing into bed with him, the tears come. I see the loss – the raw, awful decay of their bond. I lose the anchor of my self-righteous anger. How can I tell her to leave him? How will I bear it when she does? I defend a position I believe he would have held when he was as young and arrogant as I am now. Still I know the certainty, the pure idealism, of that man are not the reality of this man.

Perhaps the arrogance of that man could only yield to the suffering of this man. Perhaps this suffering is more real than that arrogance. Perhaps I should honor this suffering.

Why don't I beg her to remain with him until the final ember of his consciousness becomes at last an ash? Do I betray him in my determination to set her free?

It is not my decision. I can't see into their secret bond. I can't know what holds them together any more than I could ever guess what brought them together. I came between them once, as all first-born children do. Still, I try to create a triangle. Now I find myself speaking with Leonard's harsh, idealistic voice, insisting that "no person should sacrifice the brief pleasures of life for another person." She must have defied him as she defies me when I try to impose my solution on her problems.

Perhaps the preservation of this marriage is more important than the quality of one life. Perhaps her sacrifice and anger and her self-pity and her rage are more than her freedom would ever be. Perhaps she *is* the marriage.

Howard Nemerov, in *The Common Wisdom*, writes, "What makes a marriage good? Well, that the tether fray but not break, and that they stay together. One should be watching while the other dies."

ALL DAY I thought it was Thursday, even though I attended a regularly scheduled Wednesday meeting. I also planned all day to attend the Annual Bar Show, which I finally realized is a week from today. After involving several people in my confusion, I had the feeling they were deceiving me about the degree of difficulty and embarrassment I cause them. I recall having missed a presentation for the Math-Science Day last Saturday, of drinking a leisurely cup of coffee at my kitchen table in my nightgown at the very time I was scheduled to speak.

If I forget the slightest thing, I am terrified. I watched a movie on television, totally distracted by my inability to remember the name of Faye Dunaway, the star. When I was surprised by the sudden recollection, it was as though I had an omen of health and sustained wisdom. Both the fear and the elation take on qualities of obsession. I have no way of knowing if my forgetfulness is the result of inattention, stress, or normal aging. Yet I am so fearful of losing a retrieved word or fact, I feel compelled to make lists.

My work is stressful. I concentrate with total absorption on the difficulties of many students. I feel engaged when I do this. I do not feel that I "drift off" inappropriately when connection is important. Although I believe that I have the ability to see into a person's reality with sensitivity, I wonder if this is a delusion.

I come out of the closet of silence as I have on other issues pertaining to the stereotyped and disadvantaged. When I say, by way of prefacing a description of my vacation plans, "My father has lost his mind," I realize that I want to wear his stigma as my badge. I want his suffering made public. Yet I know it is a badge I may never be able to discard. Claiming my father's illness may mean embracing the possible genetic link.

I SIT ON THE STAGE during the commencement ceremony. While my academic regalia is too warm and somewhat uncomfortable, I experience the recurrent amazement of finding myself on this side of the proscenium. I think, as I always do, on this or similar occasions, of how proud he would be to see me sitting on the stage, representing the dean and the college, and the ideals I learned by his example.

Near the top of the field house, I see a faculty member who retired just this past December, a man whose resemblance to my father attracted my attention years ago when I took accounting from him at another university. He retired after several awkward years during which increasing numbers of students complained about his incoherence and forgetfulness. He is a man who was once feared by students subjected to his intellectual rigor. Prior to his forced retirement, he was ridiculed by students who could not make sense of his lectures, and who realized that he was writing nonsense on the blackboard.

I am chilled by premonition, as though he is the ghost of future commencements. Do I love this ritual so dearly that I will still come to watch the ceremonies of colleagues after they have been forced to evict me from their ranks?

By coming out of the closet of fear, do I risk accelerating the eviction process? Do I forewarn the colleagues who will evaluate my performance, who will gather anecdotes, who will compare notes, who will reduce my teaching responsibilities, who will withhold raises, who will not respect or accept me anymore?

*W*E LEAVE CALIFORNIA *after World War II because there will not be enough work for everyone, and because it is important to return to a simple, pastoral life. If the worst were to happen, those who had the foresight to return to the land would have the advantage over those who had remained dependent upon technology and an uncertain job market.*

We spend almost two years living with Nana and Grandad before Daddy buys the farm. The purchase of the farm is the realization of his pastoral dream. The farm will set us apart from ordinary people at a time in my life when I care only about conformity.

I am furious with Daddy for ruining my life by moving from California. When he moves us to the farm, I feel as though he is sealing me into a coffin. I belong on the beach. I long for the tides and the horizon of the Pacific. I have no pioneer spirit. I dread being confined to a small farm outside a small town in Kansas.

His zeal is boundless. The farmhouse is an abandoned country club facing an empty lake bottom by a broken dam. The lake bottom is a jungle of weeds that we are to conquer with a Ford tractor and a plow. We must each take our turn with the mowing and then the plowing of the dense stubble.

I suffer the monotony of the slow circles the plow makes, trying to dramatize the experience. I sing. I recite poetry I memorize especially so I will have the material for solitude. I fantasize endlessly about love, changing from one leading man to another, having become acutely aware of the contrast between small-town boys and farm boys and beach boys. I'm hypnotized by the heat and the rhythm of the plow against the tide of the furrows of the field.

I am startled from my trance by a small, shrill squeak behind me. I turn to see the severed body of a bright and furry baby rabbit swept aside by the blade of the plow. Then, from nowhere, baby rabbits are scattering everywhere. Before I can find the gearshift or the key to stop the engine, the plow has mutilated two, perhaps three or more, baby rabbits.

I'm crying as I wade through the soft waves of freshly plowed earth. He is running across the field to meet me, certain, I know, that I am injured. We meet, heaving and shaking. His eyes are piercing in his pale face.

"I've killed them. Oh, how many, Oh, the baby . . . "

"Rabbits? Only rabbits? I thought you were hurt."

"I couldn't stop in time. I . . . "

He sets his jaw. "You couldn't kill all the rabbits on this farm with a plow even if you tried. The world would be overrun with rabbits if none were killed."

"I'm not going to plow anymore."

"Now, listen here, young lady. The only way to clear that lake bottom is to plow it. The rabbits will find other places to nest."

"But I won't kill them. You can't make me."

"You are going to take your turn plowing. Enough of this sentiment."

I plow. I do not speak to him for three days. Finally, he puts his copy of The Origin of Species by my bedside table. After a few weeks, he joins me on the bank of the stream and tells me how an understanding of science and of principles such as that of natural selection or survival of the fittest make life more understandable.

He concludes his lecture, which I have heard in icy silence, with words to the effect that "when we see ourselves and our own lives as relatively unimportant in the grand scheme of things, we can let go of the impulse to suffer needlessly."

Perhaps the plow saved the rabbits from the coyote we hear beyond the evening music of the cicadas.

S HE TELLS ME that he is sitting at the kitchen counter eating
cones without ice cream. Although there is ice cream in the
freezer, she doesn't get it for him, or point out his omission to
him.

She has her passport for the European tour. When the passport
arrived, she explained to Daddy that she had sent for a passport so
she would have one if she ever needed it. He had responded,
"That's a good idea."

She has misgivings. I take her through "the worst thing that
could happen" exercise. He could die while she is gone. She will
leave the telephone number of the San Diego research group that
will do the autopsy. "He could fall, and die from the fall," she says.
Or, "He could fall and not be seriously injured." Then he would
have to be taken to the hospital. Tom could manage his admission
by phone, or, within a few hours, in person. I could fly there to
help if it were serious enough. She decides not to buy the insurance that guarantees a flight home at the charter rate for a passenger called home by an emergency. In the case of an emergency too
serious for the hired caregiver, we could attempt to have him admitted to Bright Haven.

We both wonder if the emergencies we rehearse are projected
wishes. Do we bury him in our minds because we are weary of his
presence, his image, his pain?

We discuss when to tell him about the planned trip. We do not
expect him to be disappointed that he is not going, or to be frustrated that she is. We expect him to forget where she is, and to
have to be reminded. She confides that she wonders if he will be
glad to have a vacation from her.

I copy her itinerary, feeling as though I have won a war.

C AROL, WAKE UP. It's five o'clock. We must start the climb
at sunrise. Wake up, Carol. It's time for our climb."
I am anchored to the ground by my hip and shoulder permeating the

*flimsy air mattress. If Tommy is well, if his sore throat is gone, I won't
have to go. Tommy is prepared for the climb. He and Daddy have been
walking the three and a half miles from the farm to town all summer. Neither of them thought of asking me to get in shape for the climb. Not that I
would have accepted had they asked. I knew they wanted to be together.*

*"Are you getting dressed? We must start before the sun comes up. We
don't want to take a chance on coming down the mountain after the sun
sets. We can make our climb and descent in one day if we stick to our
plan."*

*"Okay, Daddy, I'm hurrying." We dress in the dark closeness of the
tent, whispering to each other above Mother's easy breathing and
Tommy's raspy breathing. I have to go. I remember how my heart
lurched when Daddy said he might make the climb alone if Tommy were
unable to go.*

*"I know you can do it, Carol. You haven't been hiking, but you have
been swimming nearly every day this summer. Your arms and legs are
strong. Your wind should be good."*

*If he did go alone, and fell off the mountain, no one would know how to
find his body. Or he could be lost. It could rain. He could be struck by
lightning. He is a "daredevil," like Nana says.*

*Tommy rouses to express his envy and disgust. I am taking his place
and he is not too sick to care.*

*As we leave our campground near the trail that will take us to the top,
he tells me to lead. "You set the pace, Carol. A brisk pace, but not one we
can't maintain. Breathe deeply. Relax. We want to enjoy the trees, the
rocks, the birds. We probably won't expend much energy talking. We
don't want to be distracted from the climb." His voice curls around the
words,* the climb, *with reverence. He has always polished certain words
so they will gleam forever in my inner ear.* Longs Peak. The climb. Our
hike. The farm. The animals. Our camp. *I shrink from this tone, as I
am almost embarrassed by the simplicity of his pleasure and his wish to
bring me into the charmed circle of his awe.*

*The trail is steep from the very start. It is seven miles to the top and
seven miles down. I know quickly how deceptive the mile becomes as we*

make our ascent into the thinning air. Our farm is three-and-a-half miles from town, but this will not be the same as two walks to and from town across gentle, undulant fields. I force myself to keep the pace I have established early on, and I try to swallow my labored breath.

"Let's take a rest. We must save our strength. We mustn't get exhausted. The hard climb will be miles from here, above the timber line." He knows I am already discouraged by my fatigue.

The bird songs become more brittle on the scarcer air. I imagine myself swimming underwater, far beneath the surface, desperate for breath, but transfixed by the sparkling mystery of the deep.

His voice is lyrical with enthusiasm. "We can stop to rest every five minutes. It's not surprising that we wear out fast at this altitude. We're experiencing an oxygen shortage."

The trail steepens as we ascend. I ask him to go ahead while I answer nature's call. I squat awkwardly behind a transparent shrub. Over my shoulder, I hear him whistling, "Oh Susanna."

Now I want to stop again three steps after our last break. These trees scrimp on their leaves, giving only sparse shelter to hermit birds who nest in their branches.

We wait to eat lunch. We time our thirst. Pace is essential to endurance. We defy fatigue, hunger, thirst, gravity, inertia. We conquer nature. We conquer ourselves. He'll not conquer me. Thunderheads gather to the north.

He promises we will stop for lunch when we reach the timber line. Then he does not want to stop. Although he has talked of "boulder field," I have been unable to imagine it. Now I see an angry, choppy sea of gray granite boulders stretching out for miles.

"Fried eggs. The painted red and yellow circles are called fried eggs," he explains. "Experienced climbers have painted eggs as they forged a trail. It would be possible to take a path which would only entrap you. All paths do not lead to the peak. Many climbers have been lost. Even climbing the west route, not to mention the east face. It is possible to take an impossible route. The fried eggs are symbols making a map to the cable. They mark the direct path from the timber line to the cable."

"The cable?" I experience a chill, and glance toward the thunder-heads.

"A cable has been installed to assist climbers with the steepest part of the climb. We will need to be very strong to use the cable." He, too, finds his glance drifting toward the thunderheads in the distance. "And to help us gather our strength, let's have our lunch."

"Shall we find a boulder on which to dine?" I ask, rising to the bait of his bribe.

He hands me an orange and takes one for himself. Each section is more than a meal. After the orange, before the raisins and nuts and cheese, he asks, "Can you imagine a more delicious meal than this one?"

"No, never."

As we eat, a moving speck appears on the horizon in the direction of the timber line. We are dismayed at the speed with which the speck becomes a man, becomes a woman, becomes an old, white-haired woman, wiry and agile as a mountain goat, approaching and then passing us with a hearty, "Good morning. Nice day for a walk." As she departs, she casts a dis-couraging put-down over her shoulder, "Do it every day. Keeps me fit."

We disregard our rule on conserving our energy for climbing. Our laughter rings in the clear noon air. We give ourselves five extra minutes of rest to compensate for our squandered energy.

When we have gathered our peels and cans into the backpack and are ready to begin again, we see the moving speck far in the distance, ascend-ing the cliff to which he has referred when describing "the cable." She moves smoothly, as through drawn to the sky on an invisible wire.

We slow to a near stop after crossing three or four boulders. He warns me to watch my step. Turning an ankle would invite disaster. The thun-derheads move almost imperceptibly.

I'm annoyed by his every word of encouragement. How can he think I will have the energy to climb the cable? I'm exhausted. It isn't fair. He isn't fair. He's always wanted me to be superior to every other person. To make better grades. To read Darwin instead of Nancy Drew. To under-stand other people's superstitions and limitations, and to never, never yield to magic in anything.

We find ourselves on a natural bridge, a ledge overlooking the valley beneath the east face of the mountain. As we sit down to rest, I am struck by the distant expanse of green. I feel the force of the green as an undertow.

"Carol. Look at me. Look up." His voice is harsh. He felt it, too. The force pulling me down. Now he asks me to examine the rock on which we rest. To his and my dismay, there is a small hole in the rock near my foot. Through this hole we can see a spot of green valley miles below the timber line.

"We must prepare ourselves mentally for the cable climb," he says sternly, distracting me from the reverie of will-lessness. We're silent as we make our way to the cliff glistening in the sunlight. We each turn inward, detached in our contemplation of the danger to come.

"I brought this rope so we could tie ourselves together. Not that this part of the climb is exceptionally dangerous. It is merely the part of the climb which requires intense concentration. We still have good energy. We are lucky. The weather has held. I was concerned a few hours ago about the thunderheads, but we know now they pose no immediate threat."

His reassurance alerts me to peril. There's no turning back. He insists on tying the rope around my waist. I recall the knot board we made in scouts. He, of course, knows knots, and Morse Code, and nautical principles, and first aid, and the names for all the muscles in the body, and how to sail into the wind when there's a storm at sea, and how never, never to show fear. Yet, were my foot to slip, were I to dangle from this thin rope, how could he hold me, how could he save me, how could he stop me from falling, with nothing but his wisdom?

Now we are tied together. He believes he could save me. I know I couldn't save him. Were his body to hurtle past me to the bottom of the cliff, what then? I couldn't survive his death alone.

We speak only of footholds, handholds. We whisper instructions to one another. He leads, controlling my pace with the slack of the rope. He moves up the wall of rock, finding toeholds in what appears to be a flat surface.

"Sorry, Carol. I've some bad news." My grip weakens for a fraction of a second. I overcorrect, gripping the cable so tightly I feel a surge of pain in my fingers.

"The cable is icy. Perhaps there is ice in the toeholds, too. This is really late in the season for a climb. There must have been frost at this altitude last night."

I feel a flood of adrenaline surging in my arms and legs.

"Our only enemy is distraction. We must do what we talked about doing. We must concentrate."

I still do not find my voice.

"Carol. Listen. We can do it. The cable is only partially icy. We're tied together. I'll warn you of the ice. Follow my instructions. Let's go."

Now I know the strength I've gained in my arms through swimming. When my toe has the merest ledge upon which to balance, I carry my weight with my arms. My hands warm the cable as I climb. I look upward, memorizing each toehold his foot leaves behind, so that my toes may more easily search them out.

We move slowly, steadily. Now we're truly beyond fatigue. We can only move upward. We could never reverse our course. Each time I shift and raise my own weight, I feel a surge of gratitude. Every time the wall reveals a chink into which a foot will partially fit, my hope is renewed.

I feel connected to the rope, and to the climber who pulls me upward with his will. I feel connected to the mountain. I think of myself floating in the ocean, of letting the water hold me.

And now the cable is behind me. We are alive and beyond danger. For a wild instant, we are helpless with laughter.

On the summit, there is a book on a pedestal. "Sign your name, Carol. You are now a member of the society of climbers of Longs Peak."

I write my name with a hand suddenly calm, in surprisingly fluid script, and then, my hometown, Meade, Kansas.

"And your age," he suggests.

"Only if you write your age," I tease, knowing his dread of aging.

He writes his name in his choppy script, our hometown, and his age, thirty-five.

Then, between my name and hometown, I write my age, thirteen. As I do so, I see a look in his eyes I have never seen before.

MOTHER ANSWERS THE PHONE promptly, explaining, "I'm still in bed. He's right beside me, curled into a nice little ball, sleeping. . . . He just said, 'I'm not sleeping.' He's had trouble opening his eyes lately. He will complain, 'Fern, I can't see,' but when I explain to him that he has his eyes closed, he counters with, 'I can't open my eyes.' It's very strange. I panic, and later, he opens his eyes without effort. . . but this is new to me. No one in the group has talked about this as a symptom."

She interrupts the conversation to take him to the bathroom. When she returns, she confides, "I've had trouble controlling him this week. He moves backward instead of forward. He pulls against me when I take him to the bathroom. I know he's trying to follow me, but his impulses go awry. He's not being contrary. He can't go forward. So, I have to get behind him and push. But, my, what a struggle!"

I picture their struggle. "And I'm not good at keeping him dry," she continues. "I wait and wait when he's in the bathroom, but then nothing happens, and when I give up, he'll wet his disposable pants right after I put them on him. And they're forty-three cents each. And immediately after I change the bed, he'll wet the fresh sheets. The pants leak sometimes. I get so provoked. I can't help but scold him."

I resist repeating my suggestion to get helpers in the home or admit him to a care home. My tolerance for listening to her recitation of her trials is diminishing. I worry that she's exhausted, and that her exhaustion makes her more impatient. I know she needs to describe her life, the dailiness and tedium of these unspeakable chores. If she cannot describe them, they will be lacking in meaning. If they are lacking in meaning, her life is a void.

If I suggest, "Why don't you hire someone to come in one day a week?" she assumes I mean, "Anyone can be hired to do what you do for him." If I plead with her to take a trip, I must mean that he would not miss her. If I encourage her to hire people to assist her with home repairs and tasks, it must mean I am unwilling to spend my time helping her. If I encourage her to develop new relationships or interests, it must mean that I do not understand the impact of this devastation on her.

The disease is isolating because as a caregiver, she truly *is* afflicted in a way that others cannot comprehend. We are enemies, bound together in the rage only mothers and daughters can know. I am guilty because by the time I experience her suffering, she will be dead and gone. I fail her and blame myself for my failure. And we never acknowledge the tension beneath the surface of our Saturday telephone rites of comfort and accusation.

If I keep my silence and resist the impulse to take responsibility for what I cannot change, she will come full circle. She will have come out on the other side of the maze with a renewed determination to keep doing what she feels only she can do. She does not want to look back and regret her own failure. She wants to remain faithful to a responsibility she sees as her own.

"What if he were lost and frightened and crying, and no one he knew was there to comfort him? What if they heard him crying and did not respond? What if he were frightened and had forgotten how to cry?"

HE WAS ALWAYS RATIONAL, never sentimental. He considered himself mortal, expendable. We were to give his body to science. We were to dispose of his remains. We were, none of us, to allow life, either his or our own, to be prolonged beyond productive, functional roles. Perhaps there are families that allow individuals to make their own decisions on such matters. For most of my life, I felt that our family was set apart because of the clarity and sternness of some of these values.

The legacy of this clarity is guilt. It is as though we are forcing him to violate his own code by permitting him to live in this less-than-human state. In one fantasy, I smother him with a pillow. His arms and legs are rigid, curled into the now-familiar fetal position of sleep. His body tenses, but he does not waken. I readily admit my crime, and I am tried and imprisoned. I serve my sentence with stoicism. I have done my father's will, knowing I have proven myself worthy to be his daughter. I fantasize myself as the living embodiment of his values.

In another fantasy, Tommy and I poison his cereal with potassium. He is delighted with the fresh strawberries and eats rapidly, eyes aglow. He is dead in moments. We dissimulate. Mother believes the disease has reached a vital part of his brain. The fantasy culminates with all of us gathered at the helm of a boat, casting his ashes onto the swelling waves on a bright, warm day. We are filled with serenity. The ghost of the bright, agile man resurrects itself in our minds. We recall his leaning away from the billowing sail of the family boat, shouting orders into the spray-laden wind, thrilling to danger.

THE PROGRESSION OF THE disease is not steady. There are odd remissions that kindle hope and memory. Mother tells of hearing his voice one night after she went to bed. She tiptoes to his door to listen. He is reciting the multiplication tables. It has been months since he has put two coherent sentences together. Now he proceeds though the sixes, sevens, and eights, like a studious and conscientious child preparing for an examination. She waits until he is through, and gives him some simple addition and subtraction problems.

"Why, I was amazed. He was able to do so many of the problems. Aren't you surprised?" Does she imagine he is improving? Why must a miracle last more than a few seconds?

*H*E LEANS FORWARD, *slide rule in hand, explaining the principles of calculus, when I ask him a first-year algebra question. By the time he has given me the background information for his explanation, I feel overwhelmed and stupid. He's so eager to pass on the legacy of his reverence for math and science and I'm so reluctant to accept it. I hate math. I hate his enthusiasm for math; he's so sure that all higher truths are revealed only through mathematics.*

*A*FTER HIS SURGERY for the subdural hematoma, he confessed that he felt "stupefied." He would say, despairingly, "If I'm really an idiot, I can always teach trig."

Now we rejoice when he can recite the multiplication tables.

He defied sentiment by giving voice to the unthinkable. In repudiating religious orthodoxy, he sought to insulate us against superstition and pain. Now he is our demon, possessing us, haunting us, harnessing us to a glimpse of irreconcilable evil. Like Job, he cannot die. Each day brings him a darker, more unthinkable indignity.

And beyond the bent frame of this frail man gleams the iridescent image of Daddy. Now solemn, brooding eyes lost on an horizon beyond the moment, forefinger curled over his upper lip; now lithe acrobat risking life and limb; now furious, chasing me across the field and into the woods, angry and unpredictable as a wildfire. And the image of his face softening, his eyes fierce with pride as he leans over the crib. The boy becoming father. The Daddyboy.

I'M THIRTEEN, *but everyone thinks I'm eighteen. Daddy has invited me to drive to Dodge City to hear the Knife and Fork Club lecture because Mother can't go. Daddy is very solemn and strange. Although he's wearing the suit he inherited from Grandfather Norman, he looks nice, and people probably won't notice how strange the back is, particularly if he keeps facing them. I am wearing my Aunt Willa's dress, a gold and black sheer crepe with a gathered peasant neckline and a full skirt with a black waistband. The style of the dress fails to disguise my angles, my jutting collarbones and hipbones.*

I am uneasy, wearing these borrowed clothes, sharing the unfamiliar intimacy of the car with Daddy who seems to have planned a list of new topics to discuss for the occasion.

Ever since Daddy persuaded the principal to allow me to take tests and skip the seventh grade, our conversations are like classes or quizzes. He hopes I won't be like other girls. He has high hopes for me. He says I can think circles around others my age. He wants to know what I thought of Darwin. I am prepared to tell him, for I knew as soon as he laid the book on my bedside table that there would be a quiz. I say that I like to be able to think my way back through time to the beginning, and Darwin seems to have done this with innocence and simplicity. Daddy agrees that the most elegant scientific theories are often the most simple. They rely upon careful observation devoid of superstition and imagination. I feel the palms of my hands moisten with anxiety, for he expects me to have finished reading the Bible he gave me for "background," and I am only halfway through Genesis. His voice is resonant with respect. He refers to our visit to the paleontologists who worked during the early summer at the State Lake.

Later, at the lecture, we are partners in the dinner conversation. The diners at our table address questions to me as they discuss the lecture. They politely refrain from asking me how old I am or where I go to school. During a lull in the conversation, I hear the heavy whisper of a woman at the next table, saying, "... disgraceful... young enough to be his daughter." I turn to see that she is looking straight at us. Daddy seems to be more proud than amused that she has mistaken me for his date.

H E WAS UP most of the night," she says, wearily. "He was very agitated, insisting that I must take some action against the neighbors who broke into our home and stole $250,000 worth of silver. He kept going up and down the stairs, searching through drawers, looking in closets and under mattresses. He was mad at me for my indifference. I explained, 'Leonard, no one has taken $250,000 worth of silver. You know we have never had any silver in the house. Even if we had, the neighbors wouldn't break into our house. Our neighbors are all good, trustworthy people.'"

"Could you reassure him?"

"No. He wouldn't listen. At such times, in such 'emergencies,' he behaves as though he's all alone, as though he's the only person with any sense of judgment or responsibility. I almost feel as I did when we were first married, as though I know nothing and he knows everything."

"Were you angry when he made you feel that way?"

"I don't know what I felt then. Now I feel so tired. As though I can't get out of bed."

"You're exhausted. It's a month since your trip, and you haven't had any days off."

MOTHER TELLS ME that William has gone to Oakland, leaving her without any assistance with Daddy. She is defiant. "I decided I would prove I wasn't a prisoner. I would go somewhere every day that Will was gone. So I put Leonard in the van and took him to the Peninsula Center. I keep the door handles taped. Well, I noticed that the tape was loose, but I didn't think he could get out. I left him in the van and went into a store.

"When I came out, a crowd had gathered. Leonard had climbed out of the van and was standing in a stooped position, you know, the way he does. A boy had stopped his motorcycle when he saw Leonard standing there. He couldn't imagine what was wrong. Then, Leonard toppled over. And people came. Of course, no one had any way of knowing where he came from or who was with him, so they called the paramedics.

"When I saw the crowd, I explained that we didn't need paramedics. I said, 'He does this all the time. He's ill.'

"Someone in the crowd asked, 'How long has he been doing this?'

"I said, 'Oh, I've been taking care of him for years.'

"Then I looked down at Leonard and saw that he was grinning. I said, 'See, he's not upset.'

"Then they helped me put him back in the van. And I drove away. All the people stood there, watching me drive away. I could see them in the rearview mirror. I know they were amazed at what they saw, and at how hardhearted I was. But then, if they thought I was hardhearted, they might just like to come home and help me care for him."

"I wonder, why do you think he was grinning?"

"Maybe he knows his situation is absurd."

"You think so? You think he knows?"

"Perhaps he was embarrassed to attract so much attention. You know he's shy."

HE IS CAPTURED looking strong and courageous in a photograph. He defies death and gravity, standing on his head on a rock perched precariously on the crest of a Colorado mountain. The rock, cracked by lightning or split by a horizontal fault, juts over the canyon floor. The notation, written in his handwriting in white ink on the black page of the photo album, reads "Foolishness." Next to this photograph is a blank space under which is written, "More Foolishness." Who snitched the photograph of him standing on his hands on the handlebars of his moving motorcycle? No matter. Family mythology will preserve the story of Leonard moving against natural forces, conquering space and time with physical grace and mental daring.

He is athlete, mechanic, accountant, mathematician, intellect, adventurer. He teaches me that "anyone who can read can do anything." As a high school student, he built a car. He has built a darkroom in every house in which he has lived.

When I'm just starting high school, he buys land and insists that the family work together to clear the woods, build fences, convert the abandoned country-club-turned-horse-barn into a house–digging the basement, pouring concrete, installing plumbing and wiring, building rooms, hiring help only to lay brick. He concedes, after having insisted that free Department of Agriculture brochures are the ultimate instruction in all crafts, that brick laying is an "art."

Tommy and I help shovel horse manure from the room which will be our living room. Daddy's eyes are lit by that infuriating inner fire when he describes his plan for glassing in the porches, for steaming loose thirteen layers of paper, for designing cupboards, for laying tile.

I am sullen. He wants us to work together, to become a pioneer family. I hate his defiance of convention, and wish we could live in an ordinary house, on an ordinary street, in town. Vegetarian, socialist, atheist, idealist–he designs a life for himself that will undermine the givens of everyone he knows. I am torn between resentment and pity. I wonder if he is an outcast by choice or necessity. Did he ever have friends? Did anyone ever like him when he was my age? Will anyone ever like me? I don't belong in Meade, Kansas. He doesn't help me belong. He doesn't know how to belong.

He is oblivious to my inner condemnation. The farm is his romance, my prison. He meanders from task to task, never quite completing one before beginning another. We pour the concrete for the basement, wall in the kitchen, and he starts putting up a corrugated steel building. Mother and I cook in a kitchen where we store our dishes in cardboard boxes. He promises he'll "get back to the kitchen to start the cupboards when there is more time."

Mother's nagging turns to icy silence. I come home late one night to find her sleeping on the sofa in the living room. Daddy starts sawing knotty pine for cupboards the next evening, whistling "Shine On, Harvest Moon" while he works. Mother bakes a salmon and cheese casserole for supper. She is full of news, talking, gossiping, and laughing as we eat the salmon casserole and baked potatoes. The picture windows are steamy, and we are warm and close. Daddy and Mother and Tommy and Linda and me. A warm little pioneer family.

MOTHER'S EVOLUTION in radical thinking has been fascinating to me. I recall her telling Daddy years ago, "You're a socialist. Clean the toilet." The expectations of her girl-hood are like the clothes in her closet that still have too much wear in them to throw away, but would bring ridicule if worn so are kept for her own curiosity and nostalgia. She is radicalized by the abandonment and inevitable death of a man who, like so many men of his time, made many unilateral decisions, labeling them "practical," or "logical," or "our way of doing things."

The contradictions between her behavior and beliefs fascinate me. I overhear her discussing the absurdity of virginity with my adult daughters, and I am flabbergasted. She says, "Can you think of anything sillier than believing you had to sacrifice your entire life to a man just because you wanted to go to bed with him? Can you believe we used to think that way?"

She has always relished stories of exotic lives lived beyond the boundaries of her own imagination or opportunity. She gives me serial accounts of a friend's daughter's search for a husband. The woman, in her mid-thirties, has had a number of ill-fated love affairs, and, after several abortions in her youth, fears the count-down of her biological clock. She wants a man and a family, and is aggressively seeking to fulfill her goal. She has read *How to Get Married* and *Lady's Choice,* an L.A. directory of eligible men and their preferences. As Mother discusses the plight of this woman looking for a man, it occurs to me that she has more than an academic interest in the problem.

"If you were going to try to find a man to date, how would you go about it?" I ask.

"Well, I do think about that from time to time. I know it's very hard to meet men. Especially for someone my age, but Betty, the woman I was just telling you about, said to me, 'Why, you're young and beautiful. You ought to look for another man.'" She skips a beat, awaiting my reaction. "Wasn't it nice of her to tell me that?"

"Yes. And true." A truth I had not glimpsed gradually dawns upon me.

"She asked me how old I was, but I got out of telling her by changing the subject."

"Well, Mother, are you going to take her advice?"

"What do you mean?"

"I mean, are you going to look for another man?" I am surprised by the sudden tightness in my throat.

"Oh, I don't think so. I just, you know, think about it sometimes."

His liberal, generous way of freeing others from the confines of crippling beliefs becomes vivid in my memory. It is as though his young, idealistic persona speaks through me. He was a man who "never looked at another woman, before or after his marriage," according to his brother Norman, who was contemptuous of his older brother's virginity. Yet, he would not want her to be faithful to the helpless child he has become. I am sure of it. I am sure of him.

"Daddy isn't able to be your husband anymore, Mother. You can care for him, and love him, and still have friends and find some joy in your own life. He would want that."

She is not changing the subject when she reflects, "Leonard doesn't always know me. Every now and then he says something that makes sense, but mostly he isn't there."

"I know. It's as though we infuse him with our memories of him, trying to sustain his existence, but that, in reality, he has gone."

Her voice falters. "He has started talking about me in the third person when he is aware of me at all. He asked me the other day, 'What's Fern doing?' And another time, 'What are Fern's plans?' I wonder if he remembers me when I was young and doesn't recognize me as that person, or if he has simply forgotten who I am."

I come back to the subject of her loneliness. "You wouldn't have to worry about his being aware of your having other friendships. His awareness is so limited, he would never even think of your whereabouts, as long as he had someone to sit with him."

"Well," she concedes, "I thought about selling the tandem bike, but then I thought I just might find someone who wants to ride that bike with me."

"That would be great. Is there someone in the bike club, or in the Sierra Club?"

"Not that I can think of, but I have noticed an old man walking around the block. He's always alone. He lives with his daughter around the corner."

"An old man? How old? Too old to ride the bike?"

"Well, not *that* old. Just older than I would like."

"How old?"

"Oh, I'll bet he's seventy-five. And he's probably not in very good shape. But I could wait for him to get in good shape."

"Have you talked to him?"

"Just to say hello. I know he's lonely. He walks a little dog."

"Invite him in for coffee."

"I couldn't do that. There's Leonard."

A S I DENY THE SOURCE of the sound, I'm pulled to the bathroom where she slumps forward, her face stunned and pale, her thighs a surprising angle over a blood-spattered stool. The white tile walls bloom with obscene poppies of oozing scarlet. I can hardly take in the danger, the shock, the finality. "Call Leonard," she whispers. I push her head down, as though she is only feeling faint, as though I don't un-

*derstand the baby is gone, that the blood signals death, finality, danger.
The party line is busy. Mrs. Ross is talking on the phone. I hang up for an
idiotic moment before I realize I must interrupt. "Call the doctor, please,
my mother is sick. I need help, fast."*

*And Daddy is here. He carries her to my bed. He picks up the receiver
and tells Central to call the doctor. "Fern is hemorrhaging. She's in
shock. We need help here. Fast."*

*"You, Carol, stop the blood. Find a napkin." I pick it up, lay it by her
side as though she could place it between her lifeless marble thighs. He's
angered by my slowness. "You do it, Carol. Can't you see she is uncon-
scious?"*

*I place the pad between my mother's legs. I cover her with a sheet. I sit
on the edge of the bed and stroke her cool cheek while we wait for the doctor who tells us that "the pregnancy is gone, fulfilling nature's plan for
preventing imperfect embryos from developing."*

*I mourn silently for the sister or brother not to be. I've lost the child as
surely as though I had carried it in my new womanly body. Later I grow
into the slow awareness that the child I lost this dark afternoon was myself.*

L INDA AND I OFTEN TALK on the telephone right after
each of us has talked to Mother. We are a typical triangle in
that we continually exchange roles, seeking equilibrium. Like so
many sisters, Linda and I are deliberate opposites. If I ground myself on the plains of rationality, she soars in the clouds of mysti-
cism. If I play earth mother, she plays flower child.

Today I am cynical while she is optimistic. I express the belief
that life is consciousness, and the wish that his body would follow
his mind into oblivion so that Mother would be set free of her tor-
ment.

She argues, "No, I think you're wrong. I told Mother that I
wished he would just go, that I was chanting for a peaceful death

for him. And Mother said to me, 'Now, I don't want anyone hoping for his death. His life is precious. I don't want him going one minute before his time comes.'"

The teeter-totter shifts. Hope stirs and soars.

"I'm glad you told me she feels that way. That's how I want her to feel. Not hating her life. Not seeing her own life as diminished as his."

I remember the dream Mother has repeated after her earlier talk with Linda. Linda dreamed that she was in a large shopping mall. She was carrying Daddy in her arms. People stopped to admire her baby. It is Linda who can always see that his life is precious. It is Linda who with ease and grace becomes mother to her father. It is Linda who teaches Mother and Tommy and me to see the more subtle planes of existence.

*H*E WANTS TO KEEP ME *under his thumb. He wants me to be a baby. He thinks anyone I like only wants "one thing." He can't keep me from going anywhere, from having friends. I won't be like they are. I want friends. I want to be desired by someone who understands love.*

"I'm going out with Alan tonight."

"No, you're not, young lady."

"I am. I'm meeting him in town at the drugstore."

"If you were going out with Alan, he would come out here and pick you up as though you were a respectable girl. He would not pick you up in town. Since, however, you are not going out, this is a moot point. You are going to stay at home, and, since it is a weeknight, you are going to study for your classes tomorrow."

"You can't keep me in this prison."

"I can keep you here, and I intend to."

"You think you can keep me from him, but you can't. He loves me. We're getting married."

"You're no such thing. You're fifteen years old."

"You can't keep us apart. It's too late for that."

"You . . . "

"Don't touch me, you bastard. Go to hell. Go to hell."

The first blow plows into my middle, doubling me over. The next is to my mouth, which blooms hotly. His fists are everywhere. There is no escape possible. I dodge, I scream for help. My father is a raging animal, intent on killing me. His eyes are ablaze.

The night hums with the sounds of summer. The locusts sing to the cottonwoods. There are scampering footprints on the roof of my room. I am bound like a mummy in bands of pain. The slightest shift in my weight causes a searing pain in my spine. I know I am crippled. I wish he had killed me.

Toward morning, I am startled awake. My father is bending over my bed, shining a flashlight in my eyes. I realize that I have screamed. That sound came from me. He does not move or speak. He studies my face. He turns off the light and leaves the room.

The next day, I can get out of bed by slowly turning on my side and creeping backward toward the edge of the bed. I can walk at a forty-five-degree angle. I see myself in the bathroom mirror. My eyes are black. My cheeks, my neck are bruised. My lips are swollen and lurid. My mother is concerned about the pain in my back and the way I'm walking, but after conferring with him, they decide that I do not require medical attention.

I determine to become remote from him. I vow that I will never again call him Daddy.

I READ THE MORNING PAPER while I have coffee. Dear Abby has complied with a request to repeat a fable about a man who was seen carrying his father in a basket to the river. He was asked by a passerby, "Why do you carry your father in a basket to the river?" He replied, "I take my father to the river to drown him. He is old. His life is of no value." The other man says, "Be sure to save the basket. Your own son will need it one day."

Every weekend I contemplate the timing of my weekly call to

Mother. If I call Saturday morning, I am more likely to find distraction by Sunday. Yet, I may become so obsessed with her mood or her news that my weekend will be more disturbed after the call than it would have been had I waited until Sunday evening.

She is cheerful, although she is full of depressing gossip from the group therapy sessions she now attends at a mental health clinic. The people in her group are all relatives of seriously ill or disturbed individuals. She laughs when she confesses, "I know I'm in bad shape when I can only be diverted from my misery by the story of someone who is worse off than me."

She has met a man in her group whose wife has Alzheimer's disease. "His wife began getting it at forty-four," my mother says, "and she's fifty now and knows nothing. He's placed her in a care home, but he has the usual guilt."

She continues, "One couple really had a story to tell. They thought their father was near death. He was nearly comatose. Then, one day, they heard him shouting, 'I've been kidnapped!' He escaped from every home in which they placed him. He climbed over the wall at Bright Haven."

She is amused by my curiosity about people I don't know. It is not feigned interest. I have always loved hearing her reveal her reactions to the people she meets. She is genuinely curious about the lives of others. She is the kind of person who leaves the supermarket with bits and pieces of information about the bagger and the man who stood behind her in the line.

She talks about the progress of the other Alzheimer's group members, such as Maureen, the woman who spent only three years with her husband before he began showing symptoms of Alzheimer's.

"She still works. Gets up at four every morning, takes him out to breakfast, then goes on her way. He's a good-looking man, although he lost his hair from worrying about his work. She has someone come in at about three every day because he starts to worry about her coming home around then. She seems so fond of him. And she takes care of herself as much as she takes care of him. She's doing all the things she had put off doing. She had a facelift. She bought herself a string of pearls and a new ring."

I never start a conversation by asking about Daddy. Now I ask.

She falters. "Oh, Dad has been. . . oh, I don't know. He was agitated yesterday. He got up early, wanted me to get his clothes. I think he thought he was going to work."

"Was he agitated for long? Did you have trouble controlling him?"

"Oh, no. He forgot."

"There's something you're not telling me."

"He's choked several times."

"While eating?"

"No. As though he had forgotten how to swallow."

I recall the chapter in *The Thirty-Six Hour Day* in which this kind of behavior is described.

"I looked it up in the book," she says. "They eventually do that. Forget how to swallow. I gave him the Heimlich. I've had to do it several times."

We pause. We both know that this is the point in the conversation at which we will change the topic. We discuss Linda's newly discovered Buddhism. She has joined a group that chants for hours, concentrating on solutions to problems of group members.

"You know she's always had problems with the man who lives downstairs. Remember how he used to pound her floor with a broom handle when she played her stereo too loud? Now he's been doing it again. He does it when she chants in her living room. I guess her living room is right over him."

"Why doesn't she chant in another room?"

"Her shrine is in her living room."

I conjure an image of her confused neighbor. How is he supposed to adjust to chanting after Muddy Waters and Jimi Hendrix?

"Why are you laughing?"

"I'm thinking about why the Buddha is laughing."

HE WAS A NATURALIST. He studied rocks and birds and tides and stars. He loved and wished to preserve the species swimming and flying in the currents and creeping on the crusts of the planet. And he saw these creatures, including himself, as insignificant specks drifting to earth from an indifferent sky. He saw himself as part of nature's balance, rather than as the center of a drama under the direction of a panoramic producer for whom his performance had significance.

And he ends his life in terror, stalked by wild animals and vicious enemies. He is attacked, mutilated, tormented in waking and sleeping dreams of horror. All the malevolent forces he understood with scientific objectivity have somehow been loosed upon him. It is as though he is possessed by the demons he spent his life deriding with scientific inquiry. He goes backward in time, downward in consciousness.

DEMENTIA IS CONTAGIOUS. As a possible heir to a dementing disease, I keep a list of my symptoms, and wonder whether they are obvious to others. I recall, before I quit smoking, having taken a cigarette from my purse, fishing for matches and finding them, taking another cigarette from the pack, then realizing that I had a cigarette poised to light a cigarette. I became alarmed when it dawned on me that I had made this very error several times.

I recall having started to write something, only to find that I held both a pencil and a pen in the same hand. I remember reaching for the faucet with my free hand while drying my hair. I confront the awful realization that I could have electrocuted myself. I've always warned my children about the danger of electricity. Have I become a child, incapable of heeding my own warnings?

I open my checkbook and see that one entry is a meaningless scrawl. I am certain I was once incapable of such an error.

I think of all the times the students have looked at me expec-

tantly, their eager eyes reminding me that I have had a lapse. I recall Daddy's early confession that he could no longer remember
the names of his students, and that he sometimes had the uncomfortable feeling that he was repeating himself while lecturing on a
new chapter in the calculus text. I think of the stacks of elementary
math books he brought home from garage sales and second-hand
stores. Was he trying to reteach himself mathematics by starting at
the elementary level?

A speaker at an Alzheimer's conference has explained that the
disease is characterized by three stages. During the first stage, the
victim knows something is wrong, but he is the only one who
knows. During the second stage, the victim and everyone around
him knows something is wrong. During the third stage, everyone
but the victim knows. Daddy is in the last stage of the illness. Am I
in the first stage of the illness, or have I simply co-opted his illness?

I am tempted to list names, dates, places I have visited, restau-
rants in which I have eaten. I count my errors and calculate the progression of my decline. My children make fun of my lapses, my
faulty memory, then dismiss my expressed fear, assuring me that
I am no more forgetful than I have always been.

I spend more and more time searching for words that escape
me. For days, I am unable to think of a word associated with op-
pressive governments. When the word *totalitarian* comes to me, I
am tempted to write it down. But I recall the lists I discovered
among Daddy's things. He had boxes and boxes of used computer
cards on which he had lists of students' names, of assignments for
various classes, of students guilty of infractions of the school's
rules. Linda tells me that she found scraps of paper on which
Daddy had scrawled only one word over and over – the word
Alzheimer's.

I vow not to make lists. I will simply become more adept at covering my errors. On the other hand, I may have become grotesque-
ly self-conscious. I may notice errors others take for granted.

I meditate to relieve stress. I reorganize my schedule to allow more time for rest and recreation. I record my fears in my journal. I also consider the odds and think about the earliest date at which I could retire from the university. I review the goals I want to achieve before I am incapacitated. And I create a scenario in which I take my own life in the last second before I become too incapacitated to make that final decision, to express the one last act of will of which my poor father was deprived.

A FRIEND, ZELLA, tells me, "Tell your mother that I made a mistake. Cliff wanted to die at home, and I wanted to help him do it. But it was horrible. I blame myself for his addiction. When he wanted shots, I couldn't say no. I had to give in. Maybe another person could have forced him to wait, but I couldn't. And the pain and the medication made him mean.

"I could have been his wife, but I became his nurse. And you can't be both. When I became his nurse, he had no wife. Anyone could have been his nurse, but only I could be his wife. I let him die without a wife. I'll always regret that... I didn't know it then. Tell your mother. Your father has only one wife."

Mother's voice is almost dreamy as she meanders through her week's activities, arriving at last at the topic of yesterday's checkup with the neurologist.

"Dad always walked fairly well when we were there before. He was having a good day when we went for our last six-month checkup. Not yesterday. I could hardly move him. He was frozen in place. I had to get behind and push him. The nurse finally had to come help. The doctor was shocked. He told me he 'had no idea that Leonard was so bad.' He couldn't believe I was still able to manage him by myself. He examined Leonard's reflexes, and then asked to speak to me privately.

"He told me I have a right to a life, that I am entitled to a normal social life. He couldn't understand how I can cope with the physical effort, let alone the emotional strain. He said I have to look ahead to the time when he'll be bedridden, and the total care that will involve. But I told him that I look forward to that time because it will be easier than what I'm going through now. Then I'll just have to bathe and change him. I won't have to push and pull him and pick him up when he falls. He pulls against me if I try to lead him. I have to push him to get him unstuck. It will be easier when he's bedridden." I don't say anything.

"The doctor had never considered that. I guess he just thinks of the idea of this disease. The reality is too awful to grasp. A nurse might grasp it, but not a doctor." Her voice is almost a whisper.

"I asked him if he could speculate on how much time Leonard has. He said he knew of patients who had deteriorated much faster. He had a patient who died a year and a half after diagnosis."

"How wonderful that would be," I say.

"Yes. But he can't guess how long it will be. He wants me to consider care homes. He said there are some nice ones where he would get good care. And Leonard might not even notice or care that much.

"His sense of time is gone. If you saw him every day, Mother, he might not even realize how much time elapsed between visits."

"I told the doctor I would still have to go to see him every day. He said I wouldn't even have to go that often."

"I hope you'll think about it, Mother. You've given him wonderful care, but he may no longer be aware of that care."

"But what would I do if I didn't care for him?"

I picture her in the empty house, facing the empty days after the moment-to-moment demands of the recent years.

"You would start the next stage of your widowhood. And it would be hard. But maybe not as hard as what you're doing now."

"Maybe not. I don't know what I would do without him to take care of."

"Do you want to come here to live? You could find a care home

for him here. Rent your house. Leave it empty. Just come here to
see if it's time for a care home."

"No, I can't do that."

*I HAVE TO WORK at the Wolfe Motor Company every day after
school and all day Saturday. Grandad is the owner, and my father is
his accountant. He says that he's giving me an opportunity most girls
never have. I can learn all the jobs for the entire business, except for the
mechanics' jobs. I have to learn how to balance the books at the end of every day and even at the end of every month. He says the Ford Motor
Company has a very progressive system, and that if I can learn it, I can
keep books anywhere. I can learn all the parts of all the models of cars and
trucks by keeping parts inventory. It is very monotonous. I check off all
the sales of parts from all the sales receipts, marking the cards in the card
file, reducing the inventory for even the least expensive gasket.*

*This part of my work requires no thought, so I daydream, waiting for
an interesting customer to come in, living my secret life. He has no patience for my daydreaming. When a customer drives up to the gas pumps
and the bell rings, he tells me I am to "run, not walk, to the gas pumps." I
have to hurry, and I have to smile. I have to wash all the windows and
check the radiator water, the oil, and the fan belt. Then, I check the air in
each of the tires. By this time, most customers are protesting, "Oh, no,
you'll get your hands dirty. The tires are okay." But I check everything,
and then ask if they need any additional service from the mechanics on
duty. The mechanics are very busy, but this is the way we let potential
customers know that we are eager for their business.*

*Sometimes I see him watching me through a window, with a strange
look on his face. But when I ring up the sale on the cash register, he is all
business. "Don't just thank them. Remind them to come back again," he
nags, even if the license plate tells us the customers are from out of state.
"Even so," he will remind me, "travelers remember good service. You
may be the one person they remember from Kansas."*

Customers are often surprised to be waited on by a girl. I always hope they know that this is a family business, and that I am learning the entire business. He tells me, "You don't have to confine yourself to women's work. You must learn as many skills as possible. Then you can be self-sufficient." Sometimes I long to be like other girls. My hands smell like gasoline.

If I worked at the Lakeway Drugstore, I'd smell like soda flavors. I would drink cherry limeades and read movie magazines, sitting on a stool at the marble counter, waiting for my shift to start. I would have a charge account, and on payday I might buy Tweed cologne or even Tabu bath powder . . . He couldn't stand it. He hates everything "artificial." He hates for Mother to wear high heels, or jewelry, or a girdle.

He wants me to work at the garage so he can watch my every move and tell me how to be, and to see that I don't turn out like other girls, amounting to nothing. He wants me to know what boys know, and to be one of the boys. He is pleased when the mechanics invite me to join them for coffee at Tony's Cafe. He doesn't approve of drinking coffee, and he doesn't know they tell me dirty jokes—sometimes three or four new ones a day—but he assumes I'm identifying with the workers when I am accepted by the mechanics.

They let me know that I'm almost one of them when they complain about their hourly rate, and suggest that they work to pay for "the old man's Colorado cabin." He doesn't approve of Grandad's Colorado cabin either, so I tell him the mechanics need a bigger percentage. His eyes soften with a fleeting moment of respect. "You're right, Carol. They can't live on what they earn. It's not fair. I'll talk to Dad." Then, as an afterthought, "And you might mention it to him, too."

He wants only perfection in me. He doesn't know I'm wild, or, if he knows, he would rather watch me closely than risk losing his temper again.

He gives me a small motorcycle because "it provides economical transportation," ignoring the exhilaration I discover in riding with the wind and flirting with danger. I wear fringed, cutoff jeans and moccasins, whizzing past George Combs, self-appointed community moralist, who shakes his fist at my back, quoting Scripture at the top of his lungs. I thrill to his disapproval, and to what I suspect is his attraction to what he sees as my "evil" nature. He has placed stones in the form of a cross on a hillside south of town, and routinely admonishes men entering the pool hall or the Oasis, Meade's only tavern, scattering his pamphlets on the sidewalk as they enter the halls of perdition, slamming doors in his face.

George appears more and more frequently on the margins of my life. One afternoon, after I have climbed up on top of the tank of the Phillips 66 delivery truck to make sure the tank is empty, I look down to see George waving paper money and exhorting me to buy proper clothing to cover myself. "You are temptation, and you will burn!" I surprise myself when I speak in a childhood sassy voice I think I've outgrown. "Speak for yourself, you dirty old man."

No sooner am I in the building than my father is by my side, his fingers digging into my arm. "Listen here, young lady, you're not to be rude to George Combs, or anyone else. I don't care how he talks to you, you are to treat him with the respect all elders deserve."

"But, he's a . . . a fanatic."

"Yes. He's a fanatic. And you're not going to change him by answering rudeness with rudeness."

I hate him for being so cold and harsh. He accepts others for what they are, but I can earn his respect only with perfection. When I do catch a fleeting glimmer of his respect, when I learn something he considers worth knowing, I feel a surge of regret. I'm so ashamed for not being his ideal daughter, his little girl, I could die.

But I don't. I smoke. I drink. I drive like a bat out of hell. I lead my secret life. I fantasize being in a fast car, driving away from this dull place, and from his silence and blame. He thinks I sit here beside him, meekly working, but I'm not here at all. If he only knew.

I AM TALKING with two friends, and I supply the name one needs for an anecdote in an instant. "Rita Tushingham. That was her name. *The Girl with Green Eyes*, I think, was the film you're recalling." They're impressed with my instant recall. "I must not have Alzheimer's after all," I muse.

"You must worry yourself sick over that, since your mental processes have always been so odd," says my old friend, Connie.

"Yes. I do," I confess with relief. "When I remember something obscure like Rita Tushingham's name, I think maybe I'm not crazy." But even congratulating myself on an instance of recall reflects my self-consciousness.

"And then, once again, you're not with us," says Mark.

"You've observed her absences, too," says Connie. "You know, there *is* something crazy about her. Something I've called intuition. Sometimes she's there, and then she's not. And, then, when she comes back, it's as though she's been there all along. She's moved back and away, and she's taken in everything, and then when she looks again at whatever it is, she's seen parts of it no one else had even guessed were there."

"And she's right. And it's amazing," says Mark.

"But someone who didn't know her so well might think it was crazy."

"So you have seen it, too, Connie. She goes away quite often. She doesn't stay away too long, but she's really gone when she's gone."

"She's a mystic," Connie reflects. "It is strange how she needs to leave to gain a better perspective. When she reports on what she sees after the trip, you always see it better than you did before."

My friends are expressing their interest in each other through their discussion about me. While I am entranced by their romantic interpretation of my flights, I wonder if I know when I am departing, when I am gone, when I return? Are my departures failures in the brain's circuitry? Are the flights of the demented often described early on with terms of endearment by friends?

For days, I list episodes of inappropriate or inattentive behavior in the back of my journal. I count the times I forget to turn off the stove burner, and the mornings I ate cereal, forgetting that I was waiting for toast to pop out of the toaster. Fear surges through me when I discover that I have gone to work without my glasses. I walk to the wrong parking lot on the campus and backtrack sullenly, only to realize with dismay that I am talking to myself. I think of a bag lady, walking along a crowded street, talking to herself, ignored by passersby.

S UDDEN DEATH is the death of preference in a society dominated by longing for instant gratification. Most of us are impatient with the victims of slow progressive diseases, and with family members of such victims. Most family members find that they are entitled to no more than three or four days of intense empathy following the diagnosis of a degenerative disease. Then, there are weeks of sensitive and deferential treatment, followed by a conspiracy to avoid depressing topics. The newly bereaved often encounter impatience from family members and friends who have decided for them that "life must go on."

How does a family grieve the loss of a person whose body lives, and whose death occurs, as one writer puts it, "too late for grief?" There is no ritual for casting out the image of the vibrant, responsive father; the passionate, adoring husband; the argumentative, teasing brother; the respectful, yet rebellious, son.

The diagnosis confirms that a death is under way which has in many ways already occurred long before the doctor was called or before the doctor summarized his grave conclusions.

Prolonged grief seeps into the crevices of my being. I lose the wild feeling of desperate grief sooner than I would have thought possible. Grief becomes a way of seeing the world, taking on the monotony of breathing.

Then there are those moments of detachment from the flattened perception, the affective disability acquired with the years' attempts at acceptance, and in that moment of moving beyond numbness, there is an illumined moment of horror so intense, so brutal, I think I'm dreaming. I long for the morning sun and the shrill reassurance of birds in the pine tree outside my window.

I DREAM that I am at the top of a stairway in a bare building with un-carpeted oak floors and undraped open windows. Light streams in. I face my accuser, a friend from long ago whose son has been brain-damaged in a car accident. Although we do not speak, I look into her eyes and know I am accused of not caring for the child who stands beside me, holding my hand and looking up to me. I protest, still without speaking, that I care for the child, but I cannot be expected to sacrifice my life for the child. She sees through the transparency of my equivocation, and I know that she understands the limits of my loving.

Now I am holding two firm, fat babies on my knees. One is the broken, brain-damaged child. One is perfect. They are both mine, and I love them, but I want to know that I can love them and still escape.

MARILYN, A FRIEND who is studying to become a nurse, calls with a tip from her pharmacology class. Her professor has discussed experiments with a drug called Narcan that has been used to treat drug overdoses. Preliminary findings indicate that it is also effective in restoring cognitive function in Alzheimer's victims.

"I thought perhaps you would want to write it down and tell your mother," Marilyn suggests.

I hesitate, realizing once more how reluctant I am to seem ungrateful for a friend's hopeful suggestion.

"Well, Marilyn, you need to know that most doctors are not very responsive to patients who bring them information about the latest medical experiments. There are hundreds, maybe thousands, of treatments in experimental stages."

"Oh, I understand that. But my professor made it sound as

though this one is really more promising than the others."

Why do I feel like the messenger about to be killed for bringing the bad news? "I'm reluctant to ask Mother to add it to her list of questions for her doctor. He isn't terribly interested in research. He regards Alzheimer's as a progressive, degenerative, and inevitably fatal disease."

Her pause tells me that she is shocked.

"Marilyn, you're going to be a caregiver, a healer. Some doctors merely manage their patients with accepted treatment. They aren't interested in exploring new forms of treatment."

"But why does your mother allow such a doctor to treat your father?"

"She takes him to that kind of a doctor because that's the kind of doctor available to her through her health care plan. And he isn't 'treating' my father. He doesn't consider the disease treatable."

Marilyn once told me, "Carol, I think you're more angry about death than anyone I've ever known." I wonder at my need to dispel the romance of the miracle cure for a future professional caregiver. I initiate her into the secret society of the angry families of victims.

"You know, Marilyn, I don't think any of us would consent to any form of treatment that might prolong his life."

"Oh, really?" Curiosity thaws her tone of voice.

"I read in 'The National Enquirer,' or some other tabloid, that Princess Jasmin was flying her mother, Rita Hayworth, to Sweden for some miracle cure that has yet to be approved in the United States. My first reaction was curiosity. I wanted the name of the miracle drug, or the name of the doctor or the name of the hospital. There is a part of you always waiting for a reprieve, a miracle, an end to the nightmare. But there is another voice telling you the truth you don't want to accept. This is a progressive, degenerative, fatal disease. Treatment in the early stages of the disease may alleviate symptoms. I have difficulty imagining how deterioration could be reversed. Even if it could, I have to ask, how much?

Daddy is in the last stage of the disease. If his disease could be treated into remission, would he be given another month, another year, to live through?"

"Oh, Carol. I hadn't thought of it in that way."

"Well, you understand why cancer patients sometimes refuse treatment. You've told me that the treatment may be even more painful than the disease."

"Oh, Carol, I know."

"I don't think any of us would condemn him to suffering one additional day. If he could be restored to his former state of intelligence, perhaps. But certainly not to any plateau at a later stage of the disease. Why, some aspects of the progression are gifts. He used to remember his recurrent hallucinations. He would brood about them. Now he forgets in the midst of an hallucination. He cannot complete a thought. Even a terrifying one."

"I hadn't thought of that."

"Near the end, he will be beyond his suffering. Then we'll simply have the pain of not knowing him. But we won't have the pain of knowing he is terrified. The horror of the disease is that it doesn't progress more rapidly."

"So the only hope is for early diagnosis and treatment?"

"No, not that either. I wouldn't want a moment of unnecessary knowing."

"Then, we hope for what?"

"For caregivers like you to give comfort to us all."

ARTHUR KOESTLER commits suicide after suffering from a disabling disease. His wife, decades younger and healthy, joins him in death, honoring a double-suicide pact.

Buckminster Fuller is stricken at the bed of his comatose wife. She dies within two days of his death, never having regained consciousness. Theirs is a double-burial ceremony.

I see Mother, clinging to her dying husband, reflecting and expressing his suffering for him, and I think about the death bond inherent in the marriage bond.

I HATED HIM for years because he did not love me enough. Now, I hate myself because I do not love him enough. Were it not for the whish and swirl of the ghosts of his former selves, circling on smooth skates, double-backflipping in slow arcs, balancing in death-defying handstands of subtle purity on split rocks over jagged canyon floors, I might abandon the search for his vanished spirit. As it is, I am a crazed miner, lured by the occasional glitter of fool's gold. I persist in this obsessive panning for meaning, trying to discover love.

It was he who suggested I read Freud, along with Darwin and Marx, when I was thirteen. The coincidence of reading Freud, just as I was cast out of the circle of unconditional love and approval, was devastating. Freud confirmed for me that I was flawed, and verified my inability to understand the nature of my imperfection.

As I became convinced that my father had not only ceased to love me, but had come to despise me, I was forced to accept that I was innately unlovable. I would not fulfill my early promise because I was not brilliant and ethical and agile. I felt I had been misperceived, and that my early promise had been a mirage. I knew I had been an imposter, and that my pretense was now exposed. Now I was known.

I embarked upon a secret life. I came to pride myself on my ability to dissimulate. I might appear to be performing my clerical duties at work, but I was really suffering in a tragic love affair. I might appear to be isolated and ignored at school, but I was really a rebel, a wild and wanton spirit. I read everything in the public library after Mrs. Pennick, the librarian, promised that I could read the books that she kept in her censorship drawer for those who had read all the "good literature." The women in the books I read—

Anna Karenina, Madame Bovary, Kitty Foyle – were all more interesting than the classmates who had snubbed me ever since I came to Kansas from California.

I lost my sense of family belonging. I no longer felt understood, accepted, or connected. I drank. I smoked. I swore. I drove fast, rode in fast cars, and was in a number of accidents which could have easily been fatal. I sought love from the wildest boys. My life passed before my eyes more than once. I scarcely remembered Sugarplum, the good and bright child. In her place, there lived an angry, unloved, and unloving rebel.

And it was his fault. If he could not love me for what I was, I would become everything he could not love. Daddyboy was dead. In his place, there lived an angry and unloving man to whom I referred only in the third person as "my father."

I turned inward, hardening my heart against a sense of betrayal or loss, thinking, "And I will never, no, never, call you Daddy anymore."

I READ IN THE NEWSPAPER about the indictment and trial of a man in Texas charged with the shotgun slaying of his brother, a victim of Alzheimer's. He had given clear instructions to his brother to kill him. The jury that heard the case acquitted the brother, persuaded that he had carried out an act of loving kindness.

I do not discuss the case with my daughters, Jana and Jill, my sons, Jeff and J. D., or John, for I know they find my views on euthanasia troubling. I am surprised when I find the article about the acquittal posted with a magnet on the refrigerator door.

"I read the article," I venture at dinner.

"I knew you would want to know what happened," Jana says.

The conversation stalls. I see myself pressing down on his face with a pillow. Then I see myself pointing a shotgun at his empty gray eyes. I cannot squeeze the trigger.

I remember having left a burner glowing unattended on the stove this morning, and Jana's sharp tone as she said, "Mother, you forgot this burner. Were you planning to cook something? You must stop doing that." I give her false assurance that I was planning to scramble an egg for breakfast, but remember having eaten cereal.

Then I have a vision of Jana pressing a pillow onto my face, followed by a vision of the man in Texas with the shotgun poised, and of the silence of the moment when his brother knows, before the shot, before the bliss of oblivion.

WE ARE DRIVING to Lawrence on a solid sheet of ice. I have been home for Christmas vacation, and because Daddy has a Ford meeting in Kansas City, he has elected to drive me back to school. I have spent the holiday testing my inner need for the creature comforts for which I have longed, while resisting their ability to control and limit my existence. I have recited volumes of barely understood class notes, on topics ranging from Greek tragedy to the process of photosynthesis, boring Mother while eliciting a glimmer of interest from Daddy. He is always willing to respond to any cue which enables him to lead me down an intellectual path he wishes to forge through the forest of female trivial and obsessive concerns.

I have been making peace with him. I want him to know that the language of liberalism, learned at his knee, has already put me in good stead with my teachers and the more discerning of my classmates. I have, for the first time perhaps, felt positive about being set apart from others by the distinctions of having had a nonconformist upbringing. He has finally become good material—eccentric rather than annoying, idealistic rather than insensitive to the mores of those around him.

Although the peace between us is tentative, I feel a strange surge of pleasure at the prospect of spending hours together in the warm car. We speed along, ignoring by silent agreement the bleak snowfields and the icy highway that should signal to us the need to drive with care, to slow down, to acknowledge danger. We hurl ourselves toward a blank horizon in which the sky and earth blend together in white harmony, ignoring the vehicle inching along the shoulder of the highway and those with hoods buried in drifted ditches.

He is a man who knows no personal fear, who feels himself to be superior to other mortals and capable of victory in any contest. He has warned me all my life that I must take certain precautions against being like other girls or women. A Wolfe woman is more like a man than she is like other women. And part of being a Wolfe, and not being like women, is not expressing fear.

I concentrate on making eye contact with him, as he does with me as we drive. If I watch the silver thread of the highway, my stomach lurches. I have his undivided attention. It is a rare moment.

"You could change your major right now. You've had the biology class, and could go right into physiology. It wouldn't be hard for you to catch up in math. It isn't too late to make a decision."

"But I love English. I know I can write. The others would pass me up in the science and math courses in a minute. You know how rotten some of my classes were. I wasn't that good a student."

"You didn't study. You have never applied yourself. You don't know how well you could do if you would only apply that fine mind of yours."

"I know it's what you want. But isn't that because it's what you would have wanted for yourself? If anyone had even suggested that you go to medical school, you would have known it was what you wanted. Now you feel obliged to suggest it to me, so I won't be deprived of opportunities, as you were."

"I don't know that I could have done it, even if I had thought of it in time. I didn't think of it when I first started school, and then when I went back, after Fern and I married, and after we'd had you and Tommy, then I had to finish as quickly as possible. My folks didn't care whether I went to school. They certainly didn't care whether I studied in any area for which I had a special talent."

"I'm so sorry. They should have known. You should have asked them to see your potential. You know how proud they are of your education, and of your intelligence. Now they would know."

"This is not the point. The point is that I see your ability, and I don't want you to waste it. You could study science. You could go to medical school. You could be a doctor."

"But it's not what I want, Daddy . . . "

"If you don't want it, it may just be that you don't know how to think about it. You may have the impression that women teach school, that they are English teachers. You may not see how unlike those women you really are, or could be."

"But what would be wrong with being like them? You have to think about who I am, what I care about . . . " Now I plead. He has given me the highest compliment he can give. He has given me permission to study science. He has given me permission to surpass him educationally. He wants to be able to be proud of me. But I feel I must pretend to be someone I am not to earn his pride. The love I want, the unconditional acceptance I need, veers away from me like skaters on flashing steel blades.

The muscle under his earlobe twitches, and his jaw is set. He has set his sights beyond the snow-blurred edge of the world we share. Again, I lose to his well-articulated reason. Again, I must set my will against his or be consumed, controlled, tamed. Again, the contest ends in a draw.

M Y MOTHER is seventy years old. She is not here anymore. She is in California trapped in a house with a dead man in a live body. Yeats spoke of being "chained to this dying animal." I see him standing in the hallway, staring at a vision in the weave of the carpet, naked from the waist down, absurdly wearing a stocking cap, a shirt, and two jackets. Mother rages, as she used to when Tommy and I had pulled a prank like painting our trike with mud. She is furious.

It is her lot to make this man lift his feet into the trousers she holds for him. He does not understand her instructions. She cannot make him obey. "Honey, lift this foot. Like this. Sweetie, let me help you. Lean against the wall, and lift this foot. Put your hand on my shoulder. Please. Lift your foot."

I write. I read. I run. I meditate. I make soup. I drink a cup of coffee. I make a normal life. I sustain myself with domestic rituals. Then the nightmare bursts open like a boil, poisoning everything. I see the image of my mother, pleading with the rigid remnant of my father. I see that she is old. She is not the tough, sturdy woman I carry in my memory. In my fixed, habitual image of her, she is younger than I am now, and she can endure everything. She is indestructible.

Linda questions Mother's endurance. She asks me if I think she could break under the strain. She wonders if Mother could simply let go of her mind, following Daddy into the thick fog. Is it possible that she could leave us as he did, becoming increasingly vague until one day we would look into her eyes, as we had his, and know suddenly that she had passed irrevocably beyond us?

I DREAM that I am playing a part in a play. The curtains are open. The auditorium is full. I realize that I haven't memorized my part; I haven't even read it. I glance at a copy of the script which I hold to my side, away from the audience, looking for the name of the character I play. I am not wearing my glasses, and can only dimly make out the print. I find the blur of a name that might be the character I am to play. I improvise, miming gestures and stringing clichés together without knowing the plot or lines. The other actors try to keep the action going, but their faces are studies in alarm. I am exposed. I know that I am an embarrassment to everyone around me. The director, who is in the wings, gestures furiously. I look beyond the footlights to see the audience leaving. The other actors leave the stage. I am alone on the stage, but the curtains do not close.

I TYPE THE DATE at the top of a memo. October 17, 1984. Today Daddy is seventy-three years old. I want to tell myself, today he would have been seventy-three years old. I cannot escape the fantasy. If he had lived the alternative life, the shadow life which seems to mime the lived life, he would certainly exceed the amazing good health and humor of his parents who at seventy-three took pleasure in friends, in children, grandchildren, great-grandchildren, and each other.

I think of Grandad squeezing Nana's knee underneath the ca-nasta table, and then of Daddy, slender and agile, smiling and pat-ting Mother's fanny. "No woman was constructed to wear a girdle. What can be more beautiful than what is natural?" he used to say. I recall how surprised I was as a teenager at the sexual play between these two shy and circumspect people.

I indulge in the game, "If he had lived the other life, the un-afflicted life," for the remainder of the workday. I see him in my mind's eye, stacking the wood by the shed, working till the falling light of dusk brings its subtle chill. He gathers dry slender logs into his arms, and moves toward the bright window of the kitchen, intent on building a fire.

He was a man given to long silences, to slow moments of trance, to reverie. I remember mystery in the deep gaze of a young man before a fire.

When I open the back door, I am alert to John's silence. He sits at the kitchen table, cradling his coffee mug and waiting for me. For a moment before he speaks, I think about turning around, going back to the car.

"Carol, you'd better sit down." He quickly adds, "No, it's not that bad. Everyone is all right. No one died. But I'm afraid I have some devastating news." We are not married. We live together in friendship, pretending our divorce of seven years ago is final, yet he will always be the one to tell me in this solemn voice what I do not want to hear. "Your mother... J. D. called... investments... precious gems... like commodities... Crandall Investment Com-

pany... closed... Securities Exchange Commission... everything gone... house mortgaged... victim of... how she could...
now she will have to... "

I start to pace, trying to make sense of the words. He captures
me on the third or fourth pass, gathering me to him, murmuring,
"Oh, I am so, so sorry." As he has so many times after so many
telephone calls. After all those times when I knew, this is the bottom, this moment is the worst. It won't be worse than this.

"She gave her money to men who said they were buying precious gems?" I ask.

"They presented this investment plan as a special one, limited
to a few select clients. It was to pay huge returns on her money."

"And it was a fake company?"

"No, not exactly. I gather it was a real company. Yes. A real company. The SEC closed it down. J. D. said there were over two hundred calls of complaint."

"Then they had other investors?"

"Yes. I guess so. She kept giving them money, converting investments, stocks, bonds, to cash. For over two years."

"And they took advantage of her because they knew she was
alone. She told them, I can hear her telling them, 'My husband
used to be a financial whiz. He handled everything, but he has
Alzheimer's disease. Now I have to take care of everything, of the
money... '"

"Carol, stop. You don't know how they... "

"And they came to the house. Remember, Christmas, when the
courier came and she made him wait on the porch while she went
upstairs, and we were sure she was giving him money, but we
didn't, I didn't, have the nerve to ask, to meddle... "

"You couldn't have known. You couldn't have known how
much."

"How much. You said she gave them how much?"

"Carol, I told you. Everything. All the investments are gone.
They persuaded her to take a $180,000 mortgage on the house, a

three-year balloon mortgage with payments of $2,175 a month. She can't pay it. They told her Crandall Investment would pay it."

"They took her money, her house, everything? These men did this to her because she was alone and scared and innocent? Because she would believe there was some magic goddamn way to have enough money to take care of her husband if he lived to be a hundred?"

"They had other investors. We don't know that it was because of Leonard that they found her."

"She would tell any stranger in the supermarket checkout line that she was taking care of her sick husband, that she had to do it all alone. And she was all alone. We certainly weren't looking after her. Her children certainly weren't helping her make financial decisions. Her children were too damn busy telling themselves the lie. The 'strong mother' lie. 'She's amazing. She wants to care for him herself. She wants him with her.'"

"Carol, don't. It isn't your fault."

"And it isn't *not* my fault."

The clues are kaleidoscopic bits and pieces, falling first this way, now that way. Frederick Terr must be the young man she referred to as her broker, the one for whom she baked a pumpkin pie at Thanksgiving. I recall the story about her being picked up in a limousine and taken to a French restaurant. I see this scene in black and white, a clip from a forties movie, a preview of a coming attraction for a feature I intended to miss. As I recall my decision to allow her this bit of private drama, I am struck again by my accommodation through denial.

Thinking of this, I remember Daddy standing by the telephone, fumbling through used envelopes and discarded lists and receipts, warning, "There are evil men who mean to rob us. They've taken three thousand dollars. It was here somewhere. We must find the money. We must find the money."

I recall Daddy's absurd ramblings during an earlier phase of his illness. I think of the recurrent themes of money, of loss, of victimization. Every expert on Alzheimer's mentions paranoia. A person who is losing his memory loses track, loses count, loses possessions. It is inevitable that a man who, in a moment of perfect lucidity, finds all his clothes rumpled on the floor of his closet, deduces that someone who meant to rob him has tossed them there. He cannot recall that he is the careless robber, and that what he sought in the clothes hanging in the closet was his memory of himself.

While he was haunted by visions of intruders scurrying from room to room, pilfering his belongings and threatening the safety of himself and his family, she was talking on the phone. She was making arrangements for the money, investing it, making a killing.

SHE IS A WOMAN profoundly affected by childhood deprivation. Her early poverty taught her that there would never be enough of anything to go around. Her mother was plagued by unwanted pregnancies that she accepted along with other hardships. To her, babies were like drought, like debt, like clouds of dust gathering in a turbulent sky. She took what came and endured her fate. But it took everything she had to persist. She had nothing left over to give. She gave neither kisses, nor compliments, nor hope to the children she tended so dutifully.

Mother, the second oldest of ten children, worked in the fields on a farm in southwest Kansas. She helped with the little ones, did her chores, and dreamed of escape. Moving to town to go to high school was wonderful. She was filled with joy and guilt to leave her worried, uncomplaining mother behind. And to make friends with well-to-do town girls. Like Hazel, who was fast. She smoked, danced, played the piano, drove fast, and called her new friend from the farm "Dizzy," then "Diz" after the novelty had worn off and her town friends had stopped wondering at the incongruity of the friendship.

Hazel dated Norman Wolfe, who was handsome, arrogant,

smooth. She insisted that her friend come along and meet Norman's shy, studious brother. The Wolfe brothers. Night and day. But both were good catches. Hazel would say anything. She was terrible really, always trying to shock people, and putting words in people's mouths.

And Hazel and Norman were brazen matchmakers. It was surely one of them who entered her name in the County Fair Beauty Contest. But after she won—it was so silly, really, being named "the prettiest girl in Meade County"—she began to imagine how her life could be different. If she were to marry Leonard, why, then, she would *be* a Wolfe. Even though she had promised herself never to marry and live like her mother, she couldn't resist Leonard.

"I didn't *really* want to get married. He sort of forced me to do it. I tried to back out, but he wouldn't let me."

And they were married in his parents' lovely home. Her mother, still nursing her youngest baby, wrote a letter explaining that she was "so sorry to miss the wedding," but that she had "nothing right to wear to such a fine affair." In a rare moment of self-revelation, she wrote, "I must say, I am sad to think that when you read this you will be married. You seem such a child."

Money was the cornerstone of the marriage, and it quickly assumed the lead role in the drama of their lives. Leonard disapproved of his parents' lavish tastes. He saw his father as a capitalist. He knew his father would never give him anything other than the right to earn his share of the family business. He had worked to put himself through the two years of college he had completed. Now he would find a way for Fern to help him earn and save what he needed to finish. He knew that even if he persuaded his father to lend him the money, his father would charge him interest on the loan.

They decided to live frugally, to keep a budget, to save even when times seemed hard, for one never knew when times would get worse. Among their love letters, there is a slip of paper on which he has written down, in careful detail, the itemized budget for their honeymoon night at the Lore Locke Hotel in Dodge City. Although he budgeted fifty cents for a movie, he later crossed it out as an unnecessary expenditure, perhaps discovering to his delight other pleasurable ways of saving money.

He made the decisions about money while she followed his instructions. He was the kind of man who would provide, and would thereby earn control. He didn't ask her to help make financial decisions, although he always offered her thorough explanations of his decisions. He studied accounting and became a tax expert. For years, he considered Postal Savings Bonds the safest investment, reasoning that, with limited funds, security took precedence over high yield. He explained to her that he didn't need to buy life insurance, since his family was genetically predisposed to longevity. He never bought on credit. He never mortgaged a home. He saved part of every paycheck. Although he was a fervent admirer of Norman Thomas and an avowed socialist, he would remain a lifelong cynic regarding welfare programs. Although he firmly believed in the principle "from each according to his ability, to each according to his need," and was willing to lend support to those who needed it, he never expected financial aid from the state or from any other person.

He believed in, and lectured to his family on, financial independence, frugality, and responsibility. He took pride in his humble dress and simple diet, yet he became wildly acquisitive in his need for tools of self-reliance and survival. He eventually filled garages and sheds and spare closets with instructional books, woodworking equipment, camping gear, bicycles, printing presses, cement mixers, cameras, calculators, typewriters, filing cabinets, flashlights, nails, wire, string, stamps, used IBM cards, carbon paper, pencils. He brought home scrap lumber and driftwood and aluminum cans and discarded newspapers. His life eventually become cluttered with these symbols of self-reliance and self-denial. He had finally persuaded everyone around him that frugality was essential to his survival.

Fern was the perfect wife, following his example and his instructions. She scrimped and saved and made do and did without. She was never generous with herself. She made her own clothes and was thrilled with castoffs. She convinced everyone who knew her that she preferred the bony chicken parts. She believed that people who didn't shop for food bargains were not clever. She couldn't understand people who stayed in hotels when on vacation, or ate out when there was food in the refrigerator. Sacrifice was essential to her character.

When he lost his will, and then his mind, her life became a brick building with rotting wood foundations. She reluctantly and belatedly took away his car keys, his checkbook, and his income tax forms. She was liberated from a role in which she had found protection, but it was against her will and at a stage in her life when she felt incapable of finding anything but despair in her freedom. She became interesting to strangers whose casual inquiries evoked torrents of self-revelation. She became a story seeking a listener.

A "financial planner" was happy to listen to such a woman, to step into the empty decision-making role. He found it amazingly simple to offer solicitous advice, to issue instructions, and, finally, to give orders. She found, eventually, that he became impatient with her when she made simple inquiries about profit. He told her, as her husband did in those safe, happy days, "I'll take care of the money. You needn't worry about it."

WHEN I CALL, she sounds stubbornly cheerful. "I'm fine. How are you?"

"I'm stunned. I'm so sorry."

"J. D. told you what happened?"

"Yes. No. He called John. John just told me."

"Well, I'll bet you can hardly believe it."

"I'm so sorry. I know you must feel terrible."

"I didn't want them to tell you. When I told Tom, he insisted that you know. I didn't see any point in upsetting you."

"How could I not know? We all have to know so that we can help."

"Well, I don't see how you can help. I don't know that there's anything that can be done."

"Mother, you can't solve this without help. I feel so terrible when I think you've known about this fraud for four months and haven't mentioned it."

"I kept thinking it couldn't be true. I kept hoping it would be all right. I couldn't believe everything could be gone. That I had let them badger me into giving them everything I had."

"Mother . . . "

"Can you believe it? Can you believe anyone could be so stupid? That I would listen to people like that? That I would let them talk me into converting all my investments to cash, just handing it all over to them?"

"They must have done something to give you confidence. You were lonely."

"You can be understanding now. But when you've had a few days to think about it, you'll be mad. You'll hate me."

"No. You mustn't think that. I am not going to hate you."

"Yes, you are. For the rest of your life. None of you will ever be able to forgive me. That's why I didn't tell anyone when I realized what they might be doing to me. This Mr. Lewis called, and told me I wasn't going to earn any profits. That Crandall might be going under. He warned me. But by then they had insisted that I mortgage the house. They kept after me and after me, and I said, 'Why, I've never had a mortgage in my life. I don't want to mortgage my house.' It was Raymond Girard – he has a degree from Oxford and speaks with an accent, he's very refined – he kept telling me I 'could be right up there with the big boys, making the kind of return on my money they make on theirs.' They had the man from the mortgage company come to Crandall for me to sign the papers. They had a special deal for Crandall customers. His name is Mr. Gerber. He's left that company, I hear. Has his own business down in the valley."

"What did they say to you? What made you decide to take out a mortgage? Had you received returns that made you think this was a good deal?"

"Well, I hadn't received any returns. They always told me I could have whatever returns I wanted, but that I would earn more if I would let them reinvest my profits. And they were so reassuring. They said I would earn the most in the long run if I allowed them to make these decisions for me. They kept teasing me about driving the van. They'd say, 'Why, Mrs. Wolfe, you shouldn't be driving that old thing. Let us get you something flashy. A Mercedes-Benz. Anything you want. You don't need to drive *that.*'"

"The mortgage . . . "

"Well, as I said, Mr. Gerber, Howard Gerber, came to Crandall. They had the house appraised. Someone came out and just walked around it, and they said I could probably get a $300,000 mortgage on it if I wanted to. Do you think that's true? Well, anyway, they had these papers drawn up for me to sign. And I kept telling them, 'Why, I don't want to sign that. I just don't think I'll do it. I've never had a mortgage. We paid cash for our house. You tell me I've got all this money, but I don't know that I really have it. I haven't seen it.' And Mr. Girard reminded me that he had offered me an annuity anytime I wanted one. They had often repeated that offer – 'Why, Mrs. Wolfe, anytime you want an annuity, we can give you whatever you want – $2,900 a month, or whatever you need.'"

"Then they had mentioned the annuity before you took out the mortgage?"

"Oh, yes. Mr. Girard would say, 'Why don't we start getting

you an income?' but he would always add, 'Of course, we can get a
larger return on your money if you don't take it.'"

"And what did they tell you the day you signed the mortgage?"

"I said, 'Now you know I don't have enough income to pay this.
The payments have to be generated by Crandall. My husband has
Alzheimer's disease, and although I'm caring for him myself now,
I don't know how much longer I can continue. He might have to go
into a care home at any time.' And they were both reassuring.
They told me that this would be 'no problem.' That's what they
both said, 'no problem.'"

"So you believed them?"

"Well, I know it's impossible for you to understand, but, yes, I
believed them. It was strange, but I was afraid to contradict them.
It was as though they had control of me, or something. It was as
though I could only get my money back if I cooperated. I felt that I
was at their mercy. That they would only continue to protect my
interests if I went along with what they said. They, all of them, had
this way of dismissing any questions, any doubts I might have,
with their simplistic reassurances. They would remind me that
they were financial planners. That's what they called themselves,
'financial planners,' and they would remind me that Crandall had
all these jewelry stores, advertised on TV, and then, there was
'The Gem Show.'"

"'The Gem Show?'"

"Yes. A fifteen-minute television program which explained
how to invest in precious gems."

*I AM NEWLY MARRIED, and am still conscious of my own
gleaming rings. I notice my mother's naked ring finger as she rubs lo-
tion on her hands after washing dishes. I ask, "Why aren't you wearing
your rings?" She answers evasively, as though anticipating my disapproval. "Why, the diamond must have fallen out of my engagement ring.
You know how tiny it was. I was sorry when I noticed that it was gone.*

But I didn't find it anywhere around the house. I suppose I lost it in the yard or away from home. I doubt if I'll ever find it. And, then, my wedding ring was worn so thin it cracked. You know what a slender band it was. White and rose gold. Remember? They were lovely rings. It makes me sad. They don't make rings like that anymore." I urge her to have Daddy buy her new rings. She laughs, asking, "Can you imagine a man like Leonard buying one set of rings, let alone two?" I have to laugh, thinking of the campaign ahead, but I'm determined to try to persuade him to make this one important romantic gesture.

I SEE THE IRONY of all of his savings, all of her savings, now consumed by these predatory schemers, masterminds of this precious gem scam. And there are the questions. How has Mother's life come to this? How could she have been persuaded to give these men the life savings for which she and her husband sacrificed luxury, comfort, even basic necessities? In what ways was she the victim of his illness? In what ways has the devastation of her husband's disease made her the willing victim of these vultures who set out to take every cent, to leave her unable to care for a man twice cursed?

"Who are these men who have done this to you?"

"It's hard to believe, isn't it? That they could know about Leonard, and lie to me about what was happening to my money? That they used it to pay themselves, and that they knew it would mean he wouldn't have care when the time came? Mr. Terr – I think I told you that I baked him a pumpkin pie – he said he had a grandmother in a care home. He was very sympathetic. Later, Mr. Lewis told me that was a lie, that he had no grandmother in a care home. Yet he seemed like such a nice young man. He was so polite, and so interested in what I had to say. He acted as though he understood my problems, as though we were working together to be certain I would be able to solve them."

"Did he ever see Daddy?"

"Well, yes, when he came to pick me up. He saw him."

"He knew, then, what this disease does to its victims?"

"Why do you ask that? What are you thinking, Carol?"

"I'm trying to imagine him, this Mr. Terr. I want to imagine them all. I would like to meet them."

"I know what you're thinking. But don't think that way."

"I want them to know what they've done. I want them sentenced to serve time in a care home. Bathing and feeding and comforting people in the last stage of the disease."

"I know you're trying to remove the blame from me, Carol. I appreciate it. But you'll come back to knowing what I did, and hating me for it."

"You are the victim of a crime. If they had raped you, or mugged you, or burglarized your house, you surely would blame the criminals. How can you blame yourself?"

"Because I should have known better. I should have been suspicious. They told me I would make all this money. It seemed like an answer. Like it would partially make up for what was happening to Dad. I know it's difficult to understand. There is no excuse."

"There's no excuse for the way we've allowed you to be the only one responsible for his care. For years and years you've lived with a person whose mind is gone, who has hallucinations and night wandering, who is incontinent . . . and somehow we didn't realize this would affect your judgment, make you vulnerable? Who was stupid?"

*M*Y YELLOW TIGER CAT, *Taffy, is incontinent and cantankerous in his senility. Daddy sees that our family is miserable, in conflict over stained carpets, and decrees that "Taffy is no longer making a meaningful contribution to family harmony." He offers to take Taffy to the Humane Society.*

I refuse his offer, saying that I have to take moral responsibility for the choice.

"Then I'll drive."

I gather the old skinny cat into my arms, climb into the passenger seat of the van, and start to cry.

"I can't. It isn't right."

"This animal doesn't deserve to suffer. It's old and of no use to anyone. It doesn't contribute to your happiness."

"I know. I can't."

"It isn't right to sacrifice your happiness and family harmony for the prolonged illness and senility of a cat."

"I know, but I can't end its life," I say, climbing down from the van.

"I don't know why you let sentimentality dominate your moral choices. It's only a cat. It has a right to die."

Taffy dies years after this conversation, long after Daddy's mind is gone. Taffy breaks a leg by falling off a balcony one year before his death. When the veterinarian tells Jana, "We have three options," she responds without missing a beat, "And I'll discuss two of them." When I comment that the poor cat is too old and weary to drag around such a heavy cast, Jana explains that she will see that I am permitted to drag around a heavy cast if the doctors ever suggest that I'd be better off if I were "put to sleep."

H OW R A R E L Y we "sum up" another person's life, particularly when that person's identity is intertwined so deeply with ours. I recall telling college roommates or new friends who seemed likely to become more than casual acquaintances that he was "not like other people."

He was a man who believed in, and lived, the life of the mind. He was a seeker after truth, an introspective, quiet-spoken man whose reverence for intellectual discovery was exceeded only by personal humility and respectful acceptance of those traveling another path. He admired Einstein and Darwin, and his economics professor, John Ise, and the shop foreman, Orville Burgin, and the farmer and customer, John N. Ediger.

He set stern conditions for himself and for his children. He had maxims by which we were to live, but from which all others were exempt. He easily forgave the transgressions of others. He would yield if time disproved a principle by which he had meant to live. Inevitably, the more humane value took precedence over the less humane. He was stern with himself and with us, but tolerant and forgiving with others.

NANA CREATES domestic rituals to make connections between loving and hostile individuals. She instructs Grandad to start the fire in the huge brick fireplace while she lights a candle at every window in a room filled with the scent of newly cut pine boughs. She creates rites for celebrating meals in different rooms of the house and areas of the yard.

We breakfast in the kitchen around the captain's table with its lazy Susan heaped with nut and fruit breads, biscuits, jellies and jams; or we have split, buttered, and broiled doughnuts with frozen grapes in the sunroom where we can observe the early morning nut-gathering activities of the fat, tame squirrels; or we have Grandad's thick pancakes and hot maple syrup on the back porch where the ivy twines to the trellis and the angel's trumpet vine climbs the old stone wall.

In winter, we have cozy lunches of buttery oyster stew and frozen raspberry salad in front of a fire crackling blue and green with magically treated pinecones. In autumn or spring, we drive to the lake to picnic on wieners and marshmallows roasted over a fire in the campground fireplace, after first gathering wildflowers or pine for a centerpiece on the camp table or quilt spread on the ground.

Suppers in the grove are often annual events—the garage picnic, the choir picnic, the family picnic. Lima beans are baked in hot barbecue sauce in huge earthenware bowls. Iva is hired to make "her" potato salad and deviled eggs, and to butter the buns and place them under the broiler at the last minute before Grandad scoops the hamburgers from over the fire in the yard. He smiles over seasons of such hamburgers, wearing any number of chef's hats and aprons with clever sayings, often offering the photographer a bite and a wink which suggests his recipe can be shared.

I feel myself nestled within this family like the smallest doll in the nest of larger painted Russian dolls. Family rituals make me feel included, surrounded by successive and increasingly mature and powerful personalities.

Yet, when I am small and my father looms larger than life, and I feel myself swept into the currents of the mystery of his tyrannical temper, I sense, above and beyond his swelling rage, the rage of his father, and the rage of his father's father.

We all become strong and distinct individuals. We each have to individuate ourselves early, or be consumed by the others' definitions of us. I am three when I know that I will do battle with my little brother, just as my father, Leonard, has done battle with his little brother, Norman. I know early that dissimulation is everything. To survive and prevail in this swarm of egos, I learn to gain attention and favor without seeming to seek either.

Grandad, the patriarch, guides us with admonitions. Nana, the mother goddess, shapes us with praise. She inevitably ignores evidence of selfishness or mean-spiritedness, seeing only our perfection. If we see ourselves revealed in Grandad's warnings as flawed, we see ourselves redeemed by Nana's grace. We are like other families in that the heritage of our men is despair and the heritage of our women is hope. We are like other families in that the fathers look upon their daughters, spirits of their flesh, and call them fallen, see them as damned.

H E IS SITTING UP when I arrive, wearing plaid Bermuda shorts and a print sports shirt. I bend down, touching a shoulder thinner and more angular than I remember. His eyes are penetrating, signifying the presence of a self.

"Hi, Daddy."

"Hi, Carol." A whisper. A flicker of knowing. Then his slate-blue eyes are again opaque.

I call Tom.

"Come upstairs, Tom. He knew me. For the first time in more than two years. Come quick. Maybe he'll know you, too."

Tom leans over, touching his hand.

"Hi, Dad. It's Tom, your son."

The intensity returns to the gaze. There are no words, but his mouth twitches slightly. He seems incredulous.

"Daddy, you can't believe this can be your son, can you? Tom, he thinks you're much too old to be his son," I guess.

Another glimmer, as though he is struggling to remember.

Later, we return from an errand and William tells us, "Grandad was only awake for about ten minutes. He has been asleep ever since. I couldn't wake him for dinner."

Mother goes to his room to check on him and quickly returns, saying, "Something is different. I can't explain it. I think he's had a stroke or something."

His body begins to tremble rhythmically, shuddering deeply to the accompaniment of guttural humming from the cavern of his being.

Mother lurches toward him, trying to cradle his rigid, moving body in her arms. "What is it?" she implores. "Oh, my dear, my poor darling. Does it hurt? Are you hurt? Oh, let me hold you."

After the convulsions subside, we go into the hall.

"What do you think it was?"

"A stroke. A convulsion. The next stage. A new phase."

"What should we do?"

"Should we call the ambulance?"

"His body doesn't seem to be paralyzed."

"But look at his face. Something has changed."

"Yes, there is something different."

"His eyes. Open, but unseeing."

"Could he be in a coma?"

"Oh, I think we should call the ambulance."

"If we took him to the hospital, what would we want from them?"

"To check him. To see if he is in danger... "

"Of what?"

"Of dying... of living?"

I WRITE THE LETTER to my father in what I now know to be my impression of his voice. The voice is scientific, stern, detached. "John and I are getting married. He is the youngest of eight living children of Hungarian parents from a town called California in Pennsylvania. His father was a coal miner until an injury forced his retirement a few years ago. Although his parents met in this country, they both grew up in neighboring villages in Hungary, and both came to this country in their late teens. The family is Catholic, Greek-Catholic to be more specific. John came to Kansas as a sought-after all-American high school football player. He has signed a contract with the Pittsburgh Pirates to play third base on a farm team. His family is nothing like ours, yet I love him deeply."

I don't say, "I love him. It's miraculous that he loves me. Be happy that this warm, funny, amazing stranger wants me. I don't know him. I may never know him. But if I don't have him, I will never stop hurting from his absence."

The letter from my father is typewritten and single-spaced. "You must sever your relationship with John at once," the letter begins. He says that our relationship is predicated on irreconcilable differences that will ensure a life of incompatibility. He asserts that "the Catholic Church, the most nefarious institution in the history of humanity, has played a leading role in the subjugation of women, in the overpopulation of the earth, and in the reign of superstition beyond the age of enlightenment."

He advises me to go to the library, and to start with the Inquisition and read my way backward or forward to understanding. He reminds me that

I've been educated to live a life of reason, to embrace the intellectual life, to put aside childish pseudo-religious beliefs that would not only blur my thinking, but that could actually affect my life, "since Catholics are among the few believers who allow their beliefs to influence their behavior."

He anticipates my objections by reminding me that I've created the impression that I was apologetic for the poverty and social status of John's family. He assures me that he is incapable of prejudice toward hardworking people forced by circumstance to live simply. He says that he would, indeed, "prefer that you choose a husband from such a background, for such a person could be relied upon to have solid values, but religious differences, unlike class differences, are insurmountable."

My father's warning excites passionate defiance in John. He is soft-spoken and to the point. "Your father has the right to fight for what he wants. I have the right to fight for what I want."

If John has been indecisive before, he is decisive now. I've never had the upper hand in our relationship. He's always kept me off balance. I had brazenly told him, "If you were to ask me to marry you, I would say yes." And he had finally, months later, whispered, "I told my mother I was going to marry you," to which I responded, "And what did your mother say?" "She said I could."

Now that there is a cast of three players, the dramatic tension increases. John and I have never had a conversation about religion. I begin taking instructions, mentioning this to him only when it is time to plan the ceremony. The priest with whom I study assures me that "faith often follows practice." I memorize facts, as I would cram for a quiz in a required course.

My mother informs me in a letter that my father will not attend the wedding if I persist with my plans. I write him, explaining, "I know this is the right thing for me to do. I will do it with or without your consent. I will be very sorry if you refuse to attend my wedding." I don't add, "And you will be sorry too."

I explain to the priest, "My father will never forgive me if he knows of my conversion. I can become a Catholic only if you consent to perform the ceremony as though I were not a Catholic." He reasons, after the slightest hesitation, that an Advent wedding will, of necessity, be a low mass. The ceremony can be performed in his study. He will give me First Communion before the ceremony, but none of the wedding guests need to know of my conversion.

I walk down the hill to the church for First Communion in the early morning darkness. Stars glisten above frozen branches that crack in the cold wind. I enter the warm church, afraid as I have only been before when acting out of stubborn necessity. My hands shake and my stomach lurches. The wafer in my dry mouth reminds me of the white wafer of fish food I placed on the water in the aquarium in first grade.

The waves of nausea subside only as I break into a run, heading back up the hill to the house with Father Towle's reassurance that "faith often follows practice" humming in my mind.

In the wedding picture, John and I are surrounded by a tiny, sedate group of well-wishers. My father smiles broadly at the camera, demonstrating acceptance from which he will never waver. He will never again refer to his disappointment, nor will he ever withhold praise and approval from John.

I never tell him of my conversion, nor of my rapid fall from grace. There will be Sunday mornings, before I am brave enough to tell John that I cannot be a Catholic, when he will return from early Mass to care for our children and I will leave the house in church clothes only to drive around aimlessly for an hour with images of the angry father and of the angry husband blurring in my mind.

N OW I HAVE LOST everything, and know I will never have peace. No matter what happens to Leonard, I must live with knowing I let all the money go."

"Mother . . . "

"I know what you're going to say. But it's true. I can never be happy again. I used to think it would be almost a relief for him to die. That I could find a way to live a peaceful life after I had finally let him go. Now this. Now I may lose my home. I won't have enough money to even take care of myself. I can't believe it."

"But the lawyers will help us fight this. Those people did not act in good faith. They never had any intention of helping you protect your assets, or of seeing that you made a profit on your invest-ment."

"It's easy enough for you and Tom and J. D. to tell me to wait for the lawyers to take care of it. But they don't say I'll win. They don't say the justice system is interested in what happens to those who take advantage of people like me. You can't tell me how we can put Leonard in a care home and still have enough left for me to live on. You can't tell me how to prepare to be evicted from a home we've owned for twenty years."

"I know. I can't tell you how to do any of this, but we've got to prepare for what comes. You have to be strong. We'll all help."

"If I have to put Leonard in a care home – and you've seen him, how his eyes have that different look, and he has only had a few spoonfuls of melted ice cream since yesterday – I can't make mort-gage payments."

I feel a jolt of panic. "He hasn't had any water?"

"No. I try to prop him up and put a straw between his lips, but he doesn't suck. I don't know how to give him water when he's like this."

He must be dehydrated. She must know. I know. Are we going to say it aloud, or are we going to remain passive? I remember the climb when I was thirteen. I was thirsty. We each had our own canteen. He had calculated the miles we must climb before allow-ing ourselves a ration of water. I recall the metallic taste of the cool water in the canteen cup. Sitting on the fried-egg symbol, a circle of red with a center of yellow painted on the huge rock. I recall his stern voice, urging me to move beyond the limits of endurance.

Cautioning me to control my thirst, conserve my energy, and deny my fear, he instructed me in courage. Now I cannot distinguish between courage and cowardice.

YOU CAN'T KEEP HIM at home another day. It's impossible. You can't change him alone. You can't bathe him. You can't turn him. You've done all anyone could do, but it's over. You have been a wonderful wife. No man could have had better care, deeper devotion. But now our group decision is to find a care home immediately."

"But I won't be able to afford it, now that I may lose the house."

"We'll find a care home for him first. You cannot keep him another day. Then, after we've conferred with the attorneys, the other decisions will simply have to follow."

"Maybe no care home will take him. They won't take just anyone, you know."

"Then we'll have to hospitalize him until we can find one that will take him."

"They are very particular, you know. Some want only ambulatory patients. Some don't want anyone ambulatory. It's difficult now. He may improve. He may be able to walk again."

"Mother, I doubt it. I don't think so."

"But how do we know? Now he may just be ill. Apart from the disease."

"Tell them what we know. How he is and what has happened in the last few days. We need a list of homes with vacancies. Tom will come over, and Loretta, and J. D., and we'll all go look at them together."

"No, I don't think we can afford it. If I lose the house, there won't be enough money. I'll have to take care of him myself. It comes down to that."

"If it takes all the money to provide care for him, you may live with me."

"I don't think we could live together. I don't know what it is, but it's as though I have always irritated you. I remember when you were in high school, even before that, I just couldn't seem to please you."

"We're very different kinds of people. We always were," I say, my voice wavering.

"It's as though you're always angry, and I don't know why."

"You're right. I am angry. I'm angry at our differences."

"But what is the difference?"

"I have to believe in change. As a professor in women's studies, I teach people how to change themselves, their lives."

"And you always want me to change. To be something else."

Now I don't want to evade the issue. I'm angry at her passivity, and I have to take take action on behalf of the man in the bedroom who is dying of thirst. And I feel a kind of fear that reminds me of myself as a fourteen-year-old bent on escape.

She won't back down. She says, accusingly, "Well, what kind of success do you have in getting old folks to change? Toni Grant, on her radio program, tells people who call in, 'You can't expect old folks to change. You're going to have to do the changing. If anyone changes, it has to be the children.'"

I retort, "So now you think of yourself as one of the 'old folks'?"

"See, you're always angry. It's always under the surface. And I never know why."

"I'm angry at anything that tells me you've given up. I'm angry at anything that is chipped or broken or torn or frayed."

"What? Tell me what?"

"I couldn't spend twenty years looking at that," as I gesture toward the backyard.

"I need to clean up the yard."

"And when I look at that, that broken vase on the windowsill, I want to cry."

"Here, I'll throw it away. I was meaning to repair it. See, I have the broken piece. I'll throw it all away."

"You needn't." Now I know how trivial my complaints are. I hate the sound of my fourteen-year-old voice. I hate my old grievances, and her compliance with my assault on her.

"Tell me what to throw away. I'll do anything you say."

"Those plastic flowers." I'm trapped.

"These? These flowers? Okay. And the vase? Shall I throw the vase away, too?"

"No. You don't have to throw anything away."

"But I will. They don't mean anything. They're just there. You act as though everything means something."

I am without mercy. "And you act as though everything means nothing."

In the tone of a disappointed mother, she says, "Well, it's clear we can never live together." Then she adds, "We've always had these differences, and we have learned to live with them. It would be a shame to spoil a good relationship, the one we have now, by living together."

I suddenly know we can live together, since we have finally expressed our differences.

IN JUNE, Mother knew she had lost her money. She denied the loss and waited, day after sleepless night, hoping to discover, miraculously, that it wasn't true. Her future would not, could not, be ruined. Finally, her worst fears were confirmed. Crandall was closed by the SEC. John broke the news to me on Daddy's birthday, October 17, 1984. I had cried several times during the day, wishing he would have the happiest birthday of all, wishing him quickly, mercifully, dead.

Within a month, I went to California to comfort Mother and to visit with the lawyers. The recollection of his face as I entered the room sends chills to my bones even now. That clear instant recognition after two and a half years of his not remembering me. His fragile voice was a whisper, but his words were distinct – "Hello, Carol."

And within moments, he was again the empty vessel of a man. His tiny, diminished body, bent forward like an ancient, abandoned frame house, leaning into a hostile wind. His eyes frozen, unblinking. And the hum of a stranger's moan escaping from slackened lips. His hands, gnarled into helpless fists, trembling rhythmically. I see him now, dressed in a rumpled sports shirt and faded plaid Bermuda shorts. His slender legs. His swollen, discolored feet.

I turned away, trying to abandon him in my heart. And I failed.

WE RETURN from having toured care homes, knowing that we must still offer Mother a reprieve, although none of us voices our despair that there is no way to pay for the care home, to find him moved to a smaller, darker circle of hell. Now he is rigid in a grotesque fetal position. He is unresponsive, lying in a state similar to a coma, but different. Mother returns to his room again and again, crooning, "What is it, my sweet baby? Oh, dear, what's wrong?"

"I think he's had a stroke," she says. "Should we call the doctor?"

One month after Mother's realization that she has lost the money, he will slip into the shadows. He will never feed himself again. He will speak again only one time, giving Mother a final gift like the one he had given me, rousing himself from a coma on November 15, to say to Mother, "Happy birthday," a response to her plea to "wish me happy birthday."

What is the connection between these events? By what fragile thread is this pitiful body tied to life?

Someday I may be grateful to Ronald and Michael Smith, to Frederick Terr, to Raymond Girard, to all the entrepreneurs involved in Crandall Investments. They may have ended my father's life when I lacked the courage to do so.

Not now. Now I wait for justice. I wait to see how our society sees a woman twice robbed by fate.

The disease is a brutal robber without mercy or conscience. Just as these men who have robbed her have no mercy or conscience. They sit in their easy chairs in the evening, tallying the day's profits and thinking, no doubt, of tomorrow's business scheme.

I FEEL THAT I am abandoning him when I leave. His eyes are unfocused but open. His body, smaller and empty of his presence, remains in the pose he assumed the day before yesterday. I shirk from what may be the final touch, then, yielding, kiss the cool, smooth cheek, whispering, "I love you, Daddy" for myself.

J. D. has insisted on getting up at five so that he can take me to the airport. We have not had much time together. As we drive along, we sort through our feelings. We have no way of knowing if our legal defense will be to any avail. I want to fight. I want to expose these vultures. Yet we realize the futility of throwing good money after bad. J. D. has researched white-collar crime, and has found it to be the most common, and the least punished, kind of crime.

"For all we know, they drained all her assets to prevent her taking any legal recourse," I say. "We have to fight. The only protection against futility is seeing this as a social justice issue."

"You're right," says J. D. "After I spend a few hours or days in her world, I begin to feel as helpless as Nana does. I'm pulled into that indecisive, helpless perspective. I am just like she is. We should do something, but what? What if we do the wrong thing? What if nothing works? It's the same with Grandad. I look at him, and I think, this isn't right. We can't just ignore what's happening to him. We must do something. Anything. I can't believe we just drove off and left him there."

"And you can't believe that I'm leaving town."

"No, I can't," he says. "But I know you're just like I am. That you get crazy. That you do what she does. She endures. She watches the slow, gradual decay, and knows she must learn to do nothing but wait. When you're here, you think you'll take some action. For the first day or two. Then you're pulled under. You submit."

"Yes," I admit. "You're right. I want to fight. I want to change something. I want to help. And then I lose momentum. I lose will."

"We all do. That's how I can let you leave. That's how I can leave. If I ever had permission to make a decision, if I ever knew I had the power to do anything, I know I'd do something. But that house, his illness, the family dynamic, the craziness, make me helpless."

"You think we should put him in the hospital," I say.

"Yes, of course."

"Even if they hook him up to machines? Even if they prolong his life?"

"I just know we can't decide. We can't know what he would want," J. D. says.

"Oh, but he always told me what he wanted. He always wanted to die before his brain died. He was very clear. We were never to allow anyone in our family to force life on a person who was doomed."

"Oh, you know for sure?"

"Oh, yes. That is why I feel so trapped. What is moral and what is right are so ambiguous. I still hear him giving me instructions. And I always respected his reason on ethical matters."

"But then he didn't know what it would be like for him. Then he didn't know what it would be like for us," he says.

"I know. I think of that. Mother still pretending she's giving him good care. When he's really dying of thirst. Yet none of us protest."

"Yes. I see our denial," he says.

"It must seem terrible to you."

"I just know someone has to take some action."

"You're right. Even if it is wrong. If he could know what it is to wait, and to watch, he would surely forgive us. He would have to know we had to give in to our own frailty."

"We've got to be able to live with this later."

"J. D., whatever action you take, I'll know it's right. I'll stand behind you."

"And I think Nana will, too," he says.

As soon as I have said goodbye, and have boarded the plane, I begin to feel the welcome detachment I know so well. And to know it for the lie it is, when, shortly before landing, I can barely stifle sobs that cause the flight attendant, and the passenger across the way, to look away.

When I call California, William is evasive when I ask, "How is Daddy?" He tells me that J. D. returned from the airport and took Daddy directly to the hospital.

"Did he call an ambulance?" I ask.

"No."

"But how did he move him?" The image forming in my mind is brighter, more vivid, than if I had actually witnessed the scene.

"J. D. picked Grandad up in his arms and carried him to his car. Then he drove him to the hospital."

"He carried him?"

"Yes. He carried him."

WE HAVE SPENT our first night at home, and I need to bathe my baby Jill. I read the chapter in Spock, and mentally rehearse the nurse's demonstration bath in the hospital. I arrange a thick bath towel on the drainboard by the kitchen sink, and then place a soft cotton baby towel on top of it. I arrange the Johnson's baby soap, the baby oil, the hairbrush with the angel soft brushes, the Q-tips, the powder. I mentally count the items. It is much too cold. I turn on the oven, and open the oven door. When I begin to perspire, I am ready to begin. Mother stands by, ready to assist. Daddy has the floodlight on the tripod, and is focusing the movie camera on me as I prepare to pick up the baby. She starts to cry as I pick her up. My breasts immediately start to leak in response. The warm milk soaks through the halves of sanitary pads I have stuffed into my nursing bra. I urge her green-checked nightie off one arm, and then the other, being very careful. Her collarbone was broken during her breech delivery, and her shoulders are taped to a tongue depressor.

She continues to cry as I slip the nightie over her head. Her umbilical cord is a dry, twisted vine. I am cautious, unpinning her diaper, fearing that I might loosen the cord and make it bleed. As soon as I remove her diaper, she pees on the nice clean towel. Mother is there in a flash, with a new clean towel. I remember to test the water with my elbow. It is just warm enough. She stops crying for a moment as I slip her into the water, holding her awkwardly just under the tongue depressor.

Now, she starts to cry again, squeezing her eyes shut, opening her little mouth as wide as it will go. She cries louder than I have ever heard her cry. I know I have hurt her by handling her too roughly. Daddy is zooming in at her with his movie camera, grinning at her sobs.

"Get away from her, you son of a bitch," I sob, as the tears I have been holding in escape in a flood.

He stops the camera, horrified.

"Oh, I'm sorry. I'm so sorry," I sob, as I soap her body and rinse the soap away.

He has retreated without a word. I can't stop crying. Neither can baby Jill. I dry her and oil her and powder her, tears streaming down my face and milk running down my robe.

By the time I have diapered her and pulled a clean yellow gown over her head, I hear the front door close.

"Daddy has decided to go home," Mother tells me. He didn't realize he was making me nervous, and he is sorry.

I have ruined his first few moments as a grandfather. I have said words he will never forget.

MOTHER'S VOICE on the telephone is indistinct. "Now they're tube-feeding him. They inserted this tube down his throat. They kept telling him to 'swallow, swallow, swallow,' and they were sounding so impatient, and forcing the tube. His eyes were filled with something, maybe fear, and I explained that he might not even understand the meaning of the word *swallow*. Then they asked me if I would like to leave the room while they inserted the tube. And I did. I couldn't watch.

"Now I feel so guilty about it. They didn't really ask me what I thought about tube-feeding. I know one woman whose husband was tube-fed for a year before he died. God, can you imagine? I tried to tell the doctor that Leonard still seemed to enjoy eating. Just a few days ago, he ate most of a meal. I told her that I hated to take it away from him if it was the only pleasure he had left. She didn't really explain it to me. I can imagine that it might just take a person too long to try to feed him when he can't feed himself. And they might feel they have no control over the amount he's fed. Now, they just fill him up. They regulate the amount. They can fatten him up and send him on his way. After they've filled him full of food and water, after the antibiotic takes care of the pneumonia, he won't have a 'medical' problem. He'll be medically fine."

"Oh, Mother, do you really think that's all they think of? Getting rid of him?"

"Well, that's what some of my friends would say. The hospital loses interest in a person on this kind of maintenance program. Not until he is medically dismissable will they stop treating him. Then, I must find a care home that will accept him. I hope they give me some help, but they may not."

"Just so you remember that you are not going to take him home. You cannot care for him any longer."

"You keep telling me that. As though you think I'll forget. I know what you want me to tell them. That I can't take care of him."

"Yes. That you are not strong enough to move him. He's too heavy. His body is too rigid."

"Still, when I look at him, when I hold his hand and look at his face – so smooth and untroubled, so placid and empty – he looks so sweet, so darn sweet. I think how good it would be to have him here with me, so that I could at least pat him and kiss him. I don't know that anyone at the hospital bothers to touch him. He's probably just an empty body to them."

"But, they're caregivers. I'm sure they're caring."

"Yes, they seem sensitive to the horror of it when they talk to me. Now he's in a fetal position all of the time. They ask me if he was in that position when he was at home, and I explain that he wasn't, that he might have had a stroke or some new devastation in his brain, and that he is less himself than he was. I tell them this is why we brought him to the hospital. Because he stopped being able to eat. And he couldn't drink water. They can't believe I cared for him at home."

"I can't believe it either."

"I still feel that I should have him at home. If he were at home, perhaps his time would come. As it is, they won't allow him to die. Perhaps he would have died by now if we hadn't taken him to the hospital."

"I know. I think of that, too."

"I know we might have done the wrong thing. I know some people allow their family members to starve. They stop being able to chew or swallow, and then they're just allowed to die naturally."

"I know. That's what I thought we would do. What I thought he would have wanted. I thought we would have to be strong, and resist getting help when he reached the final stage. That's what I thought before it happened."

"But how could anyone endure that? How could we live with that agony, with knowing he was dying by inches?"

"It was an abstraction. A noble principle until the time came. I know I couldn't go into his room. I couldn't watch it happen. You couldn't watch that, live with that. You've had too much."

"And yet, we may look back on this and realize that we were really wrong."

"No matter how long this lasts, we have to know that even if we were wrong, we couldn't bear his pain."

"I thought about how it must hurt. Hunger. And thirst. I know it hurts. Even if he doesn't really know anything else."

"You had to see that he had the kind of care he needed, Mother. You did what you had to do."

"I don't know how the others do it. How they let them starve. I don't believe in 'heroic measures,' and I told them at the hospital not to do anything extra, but I know they're afraid they'll be sued later, no matter what we say. They don't trust any of us. They know we're crazy from all we've been through. And they must know how we change our minds. How we wait and hope for death, and then panic when we see those haunting, glazed eyes. There is a moment so fearful that I would give anything for help. And for freedom. I want someone else to decide."

"Yes, Mother, I know. You want whatever is going to happen to just happen. And to know you're not making it happen."

"Carol, we have to remember that there might still be enough consciousness for him to know."

"What do you mean?"

"I keep thinking that he might know we are not trying to save him. How terrible for him to know how impatient we are."

I DREAM of a bright garden enclosed by tall hollyhocks. Within the garden there is a presence. The presence of the absent child. I remember the sweet, blond boy of three. When I awaken, I think it is a dream about missing Jeff, my grown son. Then I know the lost child is Daddy.

THE HOSPITAL has transferred Daddy to a care home because his pneumonia has subsided and, although his condition appears otherwise unchanged, he is no longer considered to be in need of treatment.

Linda tells me on the telephone, "I felt better about his being in the care home when I first saw him. He looked clean and peaceful, like a sleeping baby. I had the sense that he was safe and comfortable."

"Oh, I'm so glad. When I heard that J. D. had taken him to the hospital, I was relieved. I felt the right thing had finally been done. I wasn't prepared to have such a feeling. I didn't know until then how guilty I had felt, how implicated by his suffering."

"Mother and I think, and Tom agrees, that we had better be prepared to refuse treatment if he gets pneumonia again," says Linda.

"Yes. Perhaps. Or is it merely that the next crisis is the one for which you are prepared? Not this one, but the next?"

"Do you think so? I want us to agree, so we'll know what to do. Tom says we need to find a doctor who will assist us with 'benevolent neglect.'"

"Perhaps Tom is such a doctor."

"Oh, I don't think he was thinking of himself."

"And he would have to think about himself."

"He was talking about the Texas case. The man who was acquitted after shooting his brother to death. Something less obvious would be preferable."

I realize how entrapped I become in this kind of fantasy. If I learned how guilty I felt about trying to ignore Daddy's condition during my last visit, I now want to admit that I can't plan for the next crisis. I think of the way I taught myself to nap during the trauma of my children's early years. I felt called upon for endless alertness. I was exhausted and depressed by the demands of such mothering, yet I never trusted anyone or anything outside myself to guarantee their survival. I hated my own fragile omnipotence. Now I want to admit my helplessness. Daddy may suffer for years, and yet I may not be able to help end that suffering. I may not be able to help him die. I also know this is more obvious to me in Kansas than it is to Linda in California. I know it is easier to understand from a distance.

"When we visited Daddy in the care home the second day with Tom and Loretta, he was no longer peaceful. Then he was moaning."

"What do you think that meant?"

"I wondered then if he knew where he was. If he knew we had abandoned him."

The familiar, well-worn trap. "If he were conscious enough to know he was in a care home, he would be conscious enough to know how sick he is. He would understand that we couldn't care for him."

"Maybe."

"Linda, he had pneumonia. He was dehydrated. We tried to allow him to take the natural path, but we couldn't. J. D. couldn't. The one who is there is the one to decide. Our group decisions aren't binding to the one who is present at the moment."

"I know. I just wish he could have the comfort of home."

"I'm not sure home was all that comfortable."

This is an all-too-familiar conundrum. Are we obligated to care or to neglect? To struggle to maintain life, or to allow death? Will he die in his own time if we continue to intervene?

When Mother is on the line, we extend the argument, each of us changing sides, contradicting ourselves.

"He looks so tiny and helpless. They say they give him eighteen hundred calories a day, but can't answer me when I ask why he is growing so thin. His hipbones. His arms. I can hardly bear to look at him. This week, before Linda came, I would sit with him and hold his hand. Then I would sit in the lobby and cry."

"I knew this week would be hard. I know it's terrible," I say.

"I can't get over wanting him to get better," says Mother. "To improve. Yet, I know if he does improve, it will just take him that much longer to die. I want him to sit up. I want him to talk. Even if it's nonsense. I want him to be the way he was before he took this turn for the worse."

Now Linda is back on the line. "We've a busy day planned. We're going to visit him twice today. In the morning and in the afternoon. To see if we can decide how much of the time he is moaning. We're worried that he may be miserable most of the time, and that we may not realize it. He could just happen to be sleeping when we're there."

Linda and Mother want connection with any lingering glimmer of his consciousness even if that consciousness is of pain.

"I wonder if we aren't overlooking the blessing of his unawareness," I speculate. "Perhaps we needn't worry that he feels abandoned. Perhaps he has descended to a level of being more primary than we can imagine. Perhaps he moans without pain."

"No, I don't think so," Mother says. "Yesterday, we gave him ice cream. They said I could do that even though the tubes are there. He swallowed. He smacked his lips. Then, when I stopped feeding him, he resumed moaning. I think he still distinguishes between pain and pleasure."

A LL DAY, I wait for the call, watching for a light on my office phone to blink on, anticipating the receptionist's voice on the intercom.

I tell my friend, Dorothy, at lunch, "It will be today. I know it." As soon as I have spoken, I wonder how I think I know.

Forgetting the time difference, I go to sleep around midnight, conceding that I am less connected to his suffering than I thought. The next morning, the call comes from Mother.

"It's happened. Leonard died last night. They called me from the hospital and told me to come. When I got there, he was gone. They said he had simply stopped breathing. I sat with him for a while after that. It doesn't seem possible."

It doesn't seem possible. Our longing for his death dissolves in the moment. She knows and I know that this is the pain for which our rehearsals were inadequate. Our longing for his death is replaced by our longing for him.

THE DAY HIS ASHES are cast into the Pacific Ocean, we release him with a simple ceremony. Tommy reads from a eulogy he has written in which he describes a childhood moment in nature with Daddy.

"Tommy, you see, nothing is as permanent as it first seems. Even you and I, we are like this pebble. We will be here for a time, but someday, we, too, will become sand – just as the pebble will become sand. But even so, we must always remember that although this pebble will become sand, the sand that it is made of will again, in its turn, once again become a pebble someday."

I DREAM that I am looking at the sky through the transparent dome of a capitol building. I see the huge gray belly of a gigantic plane which hangs in the air six inches above the dome. I realize that I am in peril. I know that the storefronts of buildings beyond the capitol have been grazed by fire. Ultimate destruction is near.

Waking, there is a bright red spot on the plant I gave up for dead last spring. On examining it, I find that the bleeding heart plant I planted on Taffy's grave is giving birth to one bright bloom. The rustle in the ivy near the plant causes gooseflesh to rise on my arms. There is nothing there.

MOTHER'S LETTER begins lovingly. She feels herself renewed by her visit with us. She apologizes for not having spoken of the lawsuit, and outlines six points enumerated by the lawyer concerning the pending case. She doesn't want me to worry about it, and I have her permission to call the lawyer to ask any questions. She needed the time in Kansas, surrounded by family and old friends, as a reprieve from the anxiety. She will continue to work through her fear of the future with her psychiatrist, and with the lawyer. She will continue her work on the past, on putting to rest her guilt and grief with the Alzheimer's group members. She praises me for my "love of mankind" and "all the good you do."

I am startled by tears. Her gratitude and praise unravel the shroud of detachment I wear to protect me from the cold night winds of memory and regret. I am vulnerable to the chilling revelation in the final paragraph of the letter. "Iris from the Neurological Society called yesterday to tell me that the autopsy results showed Leonard had both Alzheimer's and Parkinson's diseases. I was sorry to hear it, but not surprised. It has been nine months today."

LINUS PAULING is a guest lecturer on campus. I listen to him lecture on "The Path to World Peace," awed by his gentle demeanor and his lively mind. He reflects on the history of war, alluding to the fact that "most wars are religious wars," and examines the likelihood of intentional or accidental nuclear annihilation. He appeals to the audience to insist on unilateral, radical action on behalf of peace.

He brings to his appeal the dignity of the conscientious objector, proven wise by the passing of time and the making of history. "This is a beautiful world. We should save it. We shouldn't destroy the world. Each person must do what he can." He certainly speaks from the perspective of the scientific humanitarian, the radical peacemaker who values human life above nationalistic pride or political arrogance. "Do everything you can. It is your duty to your children, to your grandchildren, to your great-grandchildren."

I resonate to his thinking with the mind of my father. I am no longer merely myself. All my life, there will be moments when I will hear his philosophy of life coming from the minds of great thinkers, and I will experience the connection to a way of thought gleaming with his precious signature.

At a dinner in Mr. Pauling's honor, I express to him my admiration for his professional and personal courage in the face of adversity. He responds as though he is surprised. "You mention my courage. Well, a lot of that may be stubbornness. I didn't like being told what to do by McCarthy or anyone. And then there was my wife. She always knew what I thought and why I worked, and I was fearful that if I let anyone keep me from my work, she would know why. I had to keep her respect."

His reference to "respect" again evokes the jolt of recognition. I know the part of him that corresponds to a part of my father. I am filled with a sense of poignancy that I can only describe as presence. For a moment, I am not bereft. I'm aware of a connection that seems to take precedence over everything else. I'm grateful for the gift of my father's contemplation and expression of noble thought. How glad I am to see these same qualities in the beliefs of another noble man.

Perhaps life is only connection. As my father left his fragile body, as he vanished behind a veil of confusion and silence, he became more vivid, more vibrant, in my mind's eye. I am startled by the realization that I am Leonard's daughter, dining with Linus Pauling, and that, although Leonard cannot know this, there is a circle completing itself in the double moment of knowing myself as discrete *and* connected. I embody his legacy of reverence for peace and respect for science. I cannot know the significance of this event apart from the pride he would take in knowing of it.

For a moment, I envision him doing a majestic double backflip beyond the prison of his decrepit body into this mystical moment of consecrated connection.

THE MYTH OF the bicycle accident injury yields its horror to a new double curse. I recall the ancient, gentle face of my great grandmother in whom Parkinson's disease caused a tremor that causes me to remember her always shaking her head in silent disapproval. I am visited by the ghost of Grandad's sister, Aunt Ada, condemned to an asylum by a husband who Nana and Grandad said "simply wanted to be rid of her," although "there was really nothing wrong with her. She could be quite normal." The ghosts of the past assemble in fragments of family lore.

I think of Leonard's intense, curious, storytelling parents in their eighties, the oldest couple in the county, honored as grand marshals in a centennial parade. The legacy of their robust good health fades with my recollection of Norman, their second son, whose addiction to migraine medication and depression eventually led to his self-inflicted death.

While it is difficult to trace a history of severe memory impairment, there are those family traits that set so many of us Wolfes apart from others—our radical preoccupation with justice; our brooding periods of contemplation and distance followed by passionate engagement in obsessive pursuits; our eccentricities that, through the generations, seem to keep others at a distance and give us material for jokes on ourselves at family gatherings.

We invent our own mythology. We are a clan. We are not like other people. We give collective testimony to Flannery O'Connor's description of a character whose age was distinguished by her becoming more like herself and less like other people.

I know I rationalize. I long to invent a bright side. Only this morning, I became so frustrated attempting to add figures from a transcript that I was rude to a student who simply wanted reassurance that he had met graduation requirements. I added and re-added figures until I had three or four totals, feeling panic rise with each new attempt, knowing the student was embarrassed by my plight, my confusion.

I recall the telephone message, retrieved from the magnet on the refrigerator, tucked into my purse as a reminder, as evidence. It is a message to Jeff, legible until the last word, which is no word at all, but jumbled letters – grim proof that I am capable of lapses in which language fails, in which the alphabet in my head collapses on its way to my fingers. I remind myself that last night I gave an hour-long speech without notes to a sophisticated audience whose eyes affirmed the conviction of my argument and the liveliness of my mind, and that last week I wrote a twelve-page article without revision, with only two typos.

I still awaken in the night with a start, as I did the first night after his death, to find my soul flooded with terror. Not sorrow. Fear. Now I think of Roswell Gilbert, the condemned murderer of a demented wife in Florida. He confesses his act, will not repent, and so must die in prison for his refusal to plead insanity. The weight falls off his bones. His lip trembles when he says, "It had to be done. Hers was no life. She lived in hell. I had to kill her. My only mistake was in not killing myself."

This case will set a precedent. There will be no mercy killing by my loving relatives in the future. The trick will be to outwit the disease, to time the suicide precisely – between the period of being able to cover faux pas and that of becoming passive. Beyond the failure to take timely action, there is the doomed life. If one misses the last moment of self-awareness, it becomes too late to choose the noble death, the death that releases the loving others from burying themselves in one's own living tomb.

Beyond these night terrors there is the sunlight of the illumined moment. Such wondrous images of the brilliant young man, vibrant with belief in the goodness of his fellows, performing intellectual acrobatics with delight in his own agility. I see his eyes alive with intelligence, his graceful, competent hands working with machines, with tools, with a slide rule... scooping maize from a pail... stroking the angel hair of the baby Linda.

It is time to release him from the prison of his illness and redeem our memory of his youth. He was a man sternly insistent on the realism of the tangible. He would not consent to the possibility of a hereafter. He was a prudent man whose legacy was rational adherence to the principles of science and of decent, responsible behavior. He wished to live a good and simple life, to cause no harm, and to do the good he could. He was extraordinary in the knowledge that he was an ordinary man. When he had given all he could give consciously, he still gave us an example of endurance, of suffering, of awful mortality.

I adored him. I worshiped him. I respected him. I judged him. I hated him. I accepted him. I pitied him. I released him.

I become him.

Carol Wolfe Konek is a faculty member in the Center for
Women's Studies and associate dean of Fairmount College
of Liberal Arts and Sciences at Wichita State University.
She was born in Meade, Kansas, and earned degrees from
the University of Kansas, Wichita State University, and the
University of Oklahoma. In addition to conducting
feminist research and writing creative nonfiction, she
works as a social activist on behalf of world peace,
women's rights, and social justice.

This book was designed
by Tree Swenson.
It was set in Palatino
type by The Typeworks
and manufactured by
Edwards Brothers
on acid-free paper.